Nonpolypoid Colorectal Neoplasms in Inflammatory Bowel Disease

Editors

TONYA KALTENBACH
ROY SOETIKNO

GASTROINTESTINAL ENDOSCOPY CLINICS OF NORTH AMERICA

www.giendo.theclinics.com

Consulting Editor
CHARLES J. LIGHTDALE

July 2014 • Volume 24 • Number 3

ELSEVIER

1600 John F. Kennedy Boulevard • Suite 1800 • Philadelphia, Pennsylvania, 19103-2899

http://www.theclinics.com

GASTROINTESTINAL ENDOSCOPY CLINICS OF NORTH AMERICA Volume 24, Number 3
July 2014 ISSN 1052-5157, ISBN-13: 978-0-323-31163-2

Editor: Kerry Holland
Developmental Editor: Donald Mumford

Gastrointestinal Endoscopy Clinics of North America (ISSN 1052-5157) is published quarterly by Elsevier Inc., 360 Park Avenue South, New York, NY 10010-1710. Months of issue are January, April, July, and October. Business and Editorial Offices: 1600 John F. Kennedy Blvd., Suite 1800, Philadelphia, PA, 19103-2899. Periodicals postage paid at New York, NY and additional mailing offices. Subscription prices are $335.00 per year for US individuals, $486.00 per year for US institutions, $175.00 per year for US students and residents, $370.00 per year for Canadian individuals, $576.00 per year for Canadian institutions, $465.00 per year for international individuals, $576.00 per year for international institutions, and $245.00 per year for Canadian and foreign students/residents. To receive student/resident rate, orders must be accompanied by name of affiliated institution, date of term, and the *signature* of program/residency coordinator on institution letterhead. Orders will be billed at individual rate until proof of status is received. Foreign air speed delivery is included in all *Clinics* subscription prices. All prices are subject to change without notice. **POSTMASTER:** Send address change to *Gastrointestinal Endoscopy Clinics of North America*, Elsevier Health Sciences Division, Subscription Customer Service, 3251 Riverport Lane, Maryland Heights, MO 63043. **Customer Service: 1-800-654-2452 (US). From outside the United States, call 1-314-447-8871. Fax: 1-314-447-8029. E-mail: JournalsCustomerService-usa@elsevier.com (for print support) or JournalsOnlineSupport-usa@elsevier.com (for online support).**

Reprints. For copies of 100 or more, of articles in this publication, please contact the Commercial Reprints Department, Elsevier Inc., 360 Park Avenue South, New York, NY 10010-1710. Tel. 212-633-3874; Fax: 212-633-3820; E-mail: reprints@elsevier.com.

Gastrointestinal Endoscopy Clinics of North America is covered in *Excerpta Medica, MEDLINE/PubMed (Index Medicus), and MEDLINE/MEDLARS.*

Contributors

CONSULTING EDITOR

CHARLES J. LIGHTDALE, MD
Professor of Medicine, Department of Medicine, Columbia University Medical Center, New York, New York

EDITORS

TONYA KALTENBACH, MD
Clinical Assistant Professor, Veterans Affairs Palo Alto, Stanford University School of Medicine, Palo Alto, California

ROY SOETIKNO, MD
Clinical Professor, Veterans Affairs Palo Alto, Stanford University School of Medicine, Palo Alto, California

AUTHORS

RAF BISSCHOPS, MD, PhD
Department of Gastroenterology, University Hospital Leuven, Leuven, Belgium

RHYS O. BUTCHER, MB ChB, MRCP
Gastroenterology and Liver Services, Concord Hospital, Sydney, Australia

CHRISTOPHER G. CHAPMAN, MD
Inflammatory Bowel Disease Center, University of Chicago Medicine, Chicago, Illinois

KAZUAKI CHAYAMA, MD, PhD
Department of Gastroenterology and Metabolism, Hiroshima University Hospital, Hiroshima, Japan

LISA C. COVIELLO, DO
Colorectal Surgery and Endoscopy, Department of Surgery, William Beaumont Army Medical Center, El Paso, Texas

JAMES E. EAST, MD(res), FRCP
Translational Gastroenterology Unit, Experimental Medicine Division, Nuffield Department of Clinical Medicine, John Radcliffe Hospital, University of Oxford, Headington, Oxford, United Kingdom

FRANCIS A. FARRAYE, MD, MSc
Professor of Medicine, Boston University School of Medicine; Clinical Director, Section of Gastroenterology, Boston Medical Center, Boston, Massachusetts

ARTHUR HOFFMAN, MD
Department for Internal Medicine, Gastroenterology and Oncology,
St Marienkrankenhaus, Frankfurt, Germany

TONYA KALTENBACH, MD
Clinical Assistant Professor, Veterans Affairs Palo Alto, Stanford University School of
Medicine, Palo Alto, California

RALF KIESSLICH, MD
Department for Internal Medicine, Gastroenterology and Oncology,
St Marienkrankenhaus, Frankfurt, Germany

RUPERT W. LEONG, MD, FRACP
Gastroenterology and Liver Services, Concord Hospital, Sydney, Australia

TAKAYUKI MATSUMOTO, MD
Department of Medicine and Clinical Science, Graduate School of Medical Sciences,
Kyushu University, Fukuoka, Japan

KENNETH MCQUAID, MD, FASGE
Professor, Chief of Medical Service, San Francisco VA Medical Center; Vice Chair of
Medicine, University of California, San Francisco, San Francisco, California

ANDREW NETT, MD
Clinical Fellow, Department of Medicine, University of California, San Francisco,
San Francisco, California

SHIRO OKA, MD, PhD
Department of Endoscopy, Hiroshima University Hospital, Hiroshima, Japan

REBECCA PALMER, MRCP
Translational Gastroenterology Unit, John Radcliffe Hospital, Oxford, United Kingdom

MICHAEL F. PICCO, MD, PhD, FACG
Division of Gastroenterology, Department of Medicine, Mayo Clinic, Jacksonville, Florida

JOHANNES W. REY, MD
Department for Internal Medicine, Gastroenterology and Oncology,
St Marienkrankenhaus, Frankfurt, Germany

DAVID T. RUBIN, MD
Inflammatory Bowel Disease Center, University of Chicago Medicine, Chicago, Illinois

CARLOS A. RUBIO, MD
Senior Lecturer, Associate Professor, Gastrointestinal and Liver Pathology Research
Laboratory, Department of Pathology, Karolinska Institute and University Hospital,
Stockholm, Sweden

MATTHEW D. RUTTER, MBBS, MD, FRCP (London, Edinburgh)
Professor of Gastroenterology, University Hospital of North Tees, Hardwick,
Stockton-on-Tees, Cleveland; Durham University School of Medicine, Pharmacy and
Health Queen's Campus, Stockton-on-Tees, United Kingdom

SILVIA SANDULEANU, MD, PhD
Consultant Gastroenterologist, Division of Gastroenterology and Hepatology, Department
for Internal Medicine, GROW, School for Oncology and Developmental Biology,
Maastricht University Medical Center, Maastricht, The Netherlands

AMANDEEP K. SHERGILL, MD, MS
Associate Clinical Professor of Medicine, University of California, San Francisco; Director of Endoscopy, San Francisco VA Medical Center, San Francisco, California

PREMYSL SLEZAK, MD
Associate Professor, Department of Gastrointestinal Endoscopy, Karolinska University Hospital, Stockholm, Sweden

ROY SOETIKNO, MD
Clinical Professor, Veterans Affairs Palo Alto, Stanford University School of Medicine, Palo Alto, California

SHARON L. STEIN, MD
Section of Colon and Rectal Surgery, Department of Surgery, University Hospitals/Case Medical Center, Cleveland, Ohio

VENKATARAMAN SUBRAMANIAN, MD, DM, MRCP(UK)
Molecular Gastroenterology, Leeds Institute of Biomedical and Clinical Sciences, St James University Hospital, University of Leeds, Leeds, United Kingdom

NORIKO SUZUKI, MD, PhD
Wolfson Unit for Endoscopy, St. Mark's Hospital, Harrow, Middlesex, United Kingdom

SHINJI TANAKA, MD, PhD
Department of Endoscopy, Hiroshima University Hospital, Hiroshima, Japan

DANIEL TEUBNER, MD
Department for Internal Medicine, Gastroenterology and Oncology, St Marienkrankenhaus, Frankfurt, Germany

TAKASHI TOYONAGA, MD
Department of Endoscopy, Kobe University Hospital, Chou-ku, Kobe, Hyogo, Japan

SIMON TRAVIS, DPhil, FRCP
Translational Gastroenterology Unit, John Radcliffe Hospital, Oxford, United Kingdom

FERNANDO VELAYOS, MD, MPH
Associate Professor, Department of Medicine, University of California, San Francisco, San Francisco, California

ALISSA WALSH, FRACP
Gastroenterology Department, St Vincent's Hospital, Darlinghurst, Sydney, New South Wales, Australia

ALISON ZARROW, BA
Jack and Maxine Zarrow Family Foundation, Tulsa, Oklahoma

HILARY ZARROW, JD
Jack and Maxine Zarrow Family Foundation, Tulsa, Oklahoma

RACHEL ZARROW, BA
Jack and Maxine Zarrow Family Foundation, Tulsa, Oklahoma

Contents

Importance of Nonpolypoid (Flat and Depressed) Colorectal Neoplasms in Screening for CRC in Patients with IBD

Matthew D. Rutter

Patients with inflammatory bowel disease colitis have an increased risk of developing colorectal cancer compared with the general population. Colonoscopic surveillance remains challenging because the cancer precursor (dysplasia) can have a varied and subtle endoscopic appearance. Although historically the dysplasia was often considered endoscopically invisible, today with advanced endoscopic understanding, technique, and imaging, it is almost always visible. The frequency of different dysplasia morphologies and true clinical significance of such lesions are difficult to determine from retrospective series, many of which were performed prior to the current endoscopic era.

Interval Colorectal Cancers in Inflammatory Bowel Disease: The Grim Statistics and True Stories

Silvia Sanduleanu and Matthew D. Rutter

Interval colorectal cancers (CRCs) may account for approximately one half of all CRCs identified during IBD surveillance. The etiology of interval CRCs is multifactorial, with procedural factors likely to play a major role. Molecular events promoted by inflamed mucosa may augment the cancer risk and perhaps explain some interval CRCs. This article reviews key studies relating to CRC risk in the patient with IBD, paying particular attention to the occurrence of interval CRCs. The most common factors implicated in the etiology of interval CRCs, in particular missed, incompletely resected lesions, the adherence to recommended surveillance intervals and biologic pathways associated with a faster progression to cancer are examined. Basic concepts for quality and effectiveness of colonoscopic surveillance in IBD are summarized.

"That Was Me" A Patient's Perspective on Flat Lesion in Inflammatory Bowel Disease

Rachel Zarrow, Alison Zarrow, and Hilary Zarrow

This article advocates the use of chromoendoscopy to detect flat lesions over the use of colonoscopy alone. The authors illustrate their point by telling the story of their father, who died of colon cancer despite following the gold standard inflammatory bowel disease protocol.

It has been proposed that effective disease control through abrogation of inflammation in IBD may also reduce CRC risk in these individual patients. This article summarizes the potential for medical therapy to reduce the risk of CRC via primary and secondary prevention, and offers practical ways in which a goal of mucosal improvement or healing may be incorporated into clinical practice.

Mucosal healing is an important therapeutic end point in clinical trials and clinical practice. There is no validated definition of mucosal healing in patients with inflammatory bowel disease, although the benefits of achieving mucosal healing include decreased need for corticosteroids, sustained clinical remission, decreased colectomy, and bowel resection. The Ulcerative Colitis Endoscopic Index of Severity is the only validated endoscopic index in ulcerative colitis. The Crohn's Disease Endoscopic Index of Severity and the Simple Endoscopic Score for Crohn's Disease are validated for Crohn's disease, and the Rutgeerts Postoperative Endoscopic Index is used to predict recurrence after an ileocolic resection.

Colonoscopy is routinely performed in patients with inflammatory bowel disease (IBD) for surveillance of dysplasia. Thorough bowel preparation is necessary to facilitate lesion detection. Patients with IBD do not have poorer bowel preparation outcomes but may have decreased preparation tolerance affecting adherence to surveillance protocols. A low-fiber prepreparation diet may improve preparation tolerance without affecting preparation quality. The standard preparation regimen should consist of split-dose administration of a polyethylene glycol-based purgative. Low-volume, hyperosmolar purgatives may be considered in patients with previous preparation intolerance, heightened anxiety, stenotic disease, or dysmotility. Appropriate patient education is critical to enhance preparation quality.

Cancer risk in patients with inflammatory bowel disease (IBD) involving the colon is high and increases with time. The quality and efficacy of colonoscopic surveillance is variable. Chromoendoscopy with targeted biopsies is superior to standard white light endoscopy with random biopsies. Although commonly practiced, the technique of random colonic biopsies has poor yield for dysplasia and has little clinical consequence. Studies have shown a limited role for electronic-based image-enhanced endoscopy, including narrow band imaging, in detecting IBD dysplasia. Efforts should focus on the dissemination of the technique of chromoendoscopy in routine clinical practice through training and quality metrics.

Patients with inflammatory bowel diseases (IBD) have a high risk of colitis-associated dysplasia and cancer. It is important that careful surveillance with colonoscopy is performed for all patients with IBD and, more frequently, for those considered to be at high risk. Traditionally, flat dysplasia in ulcerative colitis has been considered to be detectable only by using random biopsy specimens of mucosa that appeared unremarkable during endoscopy. However, recent studies have shown that most of them are visible; thus, their detection as nonpolypoid colorectal neoplasms is an integral component in the prevention of colitic cancer.

Enhanced surveillance colonoscopy techniques for dysplasia detection in ulcerative colitis have successfully been implemented into group and solo practices. Chromoendoscopy (CE), in particular, has been shown to significantly increase dysplasia detection in surveillance of patients with inflammatory bowel disease. CE can be learned and is reproducible, with an associated modest increase in procedure time.

Endomicroscopy is a new imaging tool for gastrointestinal endoscopy. In-vivo histology becomes possible at subcellular resolution during ongoing colonoscopy. Panchromoendoscopy with targeted biopsies has become the method of choice for surveillance of patients with inflammatory bowel disease. Endomicroscopy can be added after chromoendoscopy to clarify whether standard biopsies are needed. This smart biopsy concept can increase the diagnostic yield of intraepithelial neoplasia and substantially reduce the need for biopsies. Clinical acceptance is increasing because of a multitude of positive studies about the diagnostic value of endomicroscopy. Smart biopsies, functional imaging, and molecular imaging may represent the future for endomicroscopy.

 Video of Endoscopic Submucosal Dissection (ESD) of a non-polypoid dysplastic lesion in ulcerative colitis accompanies this article

Much of the flat or biopsy-only detected dysplasia in inflammatory bowel disease (IBD) that had historically warranted a colectomy can now be shown to be circumscribed lesions with dye-spray or advanced endoscopic imaging. These lesions are therefore amenable to endoscopic excision with close endoscopic follow-up, though are technically very challenging. This review discusses preresection assessment of nonpoly-poid or flat (Paris 0-II) lesions in colitis; lifting with colloids or hyaluronate; endoscopic mucosal resection (EMR) with spiral or flat ribbon snares; or simplified, hybrid, and full endoscopic submucosal dissection (ESD); as well as mucosal ablation. Close follow-up postresection is mandatory.

Patients with inflammatory bowel disease (IBD) and dysplasia have pathologic characteristics and risks different from those of patients with sporadic carcinomas. Therefore, surgical interventions need to be more aggressive than in sporadic cases. This article reviews the surgical management of nonpolypoid lesions, dysplasia, and strictures found in patients with IBD.

Patients with inflammatory bowel disease may develop dysplasia in the cryptal epithelium, polypoid neoplasias, and nonpolypoid (flat) adenomas, lesions at risk to proceed to colorectal carcinoma. The onset of invasion in nonpolypoid adenomas may occur without changes in the shape or the size of the lesion. In experimental animals, some colonotropic carcinogens induce polypoid and nonpolypoid neoplasias and others induce polypoid neoplasias exclusively. Some of the biologic attributes of nonpolypoid adenomas in humans can be demonstrated in laboratory animals.

Surveillance colonoscopy in patients with inflammatory bowel disease (IBD) with colonic involvement is recommended by multiple national and international gastrointestinal societies. Recommendations differ on the timing of initial screening colonoscopy, recommended surveillance inter-vals, optimal technique for dysplasia detection, and management of endo-scopically visible and nonvisible dysplasia. This article reviews current society guidelines, highlighting similarities and differences, in an attempt to summarize areas of consensus on surveillance protocols in IBD, while drawing attention to controversial areas in need of further research.

The role of endoscopy in the management of patients with inflammatory bowel disease (IBD) is well established. However, recent data have shown significant limitations in the effectiveness of colonoscopy in preventing colorectal cancer (CRC) in patients with IBD colitis. The current standard random biopsy seemed largely ineffective in detecting nonpolypoid colo-rectal neoplasms. Data using chromoendoscopy with targeted biopsy, however, showed a significant improvement when used to detect dysplasia, the best predictor of CRC risk. This article provides a useful and organized series of images of the detection, diagnosis and management of the superficial elevated, flat, and depressed colorectal neoplasms in IBD patients, and provides a technical guide for the use of chromoendoscopy with targeted biopsy.

GASTROINTESTINAL ENDOSCOPY CLINICS OF NORTH AMERICA

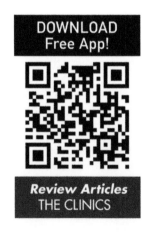

Foreword

Learning to Detect Flat Neoplastic Lesions in Inflammatory Bowel Disease

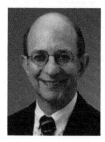

Charles J. Lightdale, MD
Consulting Editor

It has become increasingly evident that American gastroenterologists have become overly dependent on random biopsies whether in the esophagus, stomach, or colon. Times have changed. Current high-resolution endoscopes combined with large high-definition monitors can now help tremendously in locating and characterizing flat lesions throughout the GI tract, which are premalignant or foci of early neoplasia. Chromoendoscopy and new versions of digital chromoendoscopy can be additionally helpful. Nowhere is this more important than in colonoscopy surveillance of patients with inflammatory bowel disease, who have a significantly increased risk of developing colorectal cancer. For years, foci of early neoplasia have been considered too occult to detect in patients with colitis. Huge numbers of random biopsies have been recommended to decrease sampling error in an effort to find dysplasia on pathology specimens. This laborious and expensive methodology has had a low yield and little benefit in community practice and has been abandoned by many.

Dr Roy Soetikno and Dr Tonya Kaltenbach are the editors for this issue of *Gastrointestinal Endoscopy Clinics of North America*, which is devoted to the improved detection and management of early neoplasia in inflammatory bowel disease. An important aspect of Dr Soetikno's outstanding career has been the bridging of endoscopic methods between Japan and the United States. Endoscopists in Japan have a better record of detecting subtle flat GI lesions. From the earliest days of endoscopy, it is fair to say that Japanese endoscopists have emphasized visual identification, analysis, and photo documentation of small GI lesions. The colon has been no exception. Dr Soetikno has incorporated these techniques, which have become increasingly feasible with steady improvement in modern digital endoscopes. Identifying small flat premalignant lesions and early cancers in patients with colitis can be lifesaving.

Gastrointest Endoscopy Clin N Am 24 (2014) xiii–xiv
http://dx.doi.org/10.1016/j.giec.2014.04.004
giendo.theclinics.com

Dr Soetikno and Dr Kaltenbach have edited an extraordinary issue of the *Gastrointestinal Endoscopy Clinics of North America* devoted to teaching and promulgating these methods, including an extensive photo atlas, which should be an invaluable resource for all academic specialists and practicing gastroenterologists.

A generous philanthropic grant has made this issue available free online. Don't fail to take advantage of the opportunity to read and share the entire issue, which should change our approach to colonoscopy surveillance in inflammatory bowel disease.

Charles J. Lightdale, MD
Department of Medicine
Columbia University Medical Center
161 Fort Washington Avenue, Room 812
New York, NY 10032, USA

E-mail address:
CJL18@columbia.edu

Preface

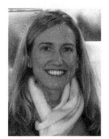 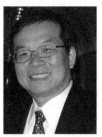

Tonya Kaltenbach, MD   Roy Soetikno, MD
Editors

It is now evident that the nonpolypoid precancers contribute significantly in the development of cancers throughout the gastrointestinal tract. Unfortunately, their detection, diagnosis, and treatment continue to represent a major problem to endoscopists. The human toll from our inability to prevent the development of many advanced colorectal cancers is highest in inflammatory bowel disease (IBD), in proportion to the number of patients undergoing screening. Therefore, the purpose of this issue is to start a renewal—*a renaissance*—in the field of colonoscopy in patients with IBD.

The challenge to a renaissance in endoscopic imaging is significant because of the seed that was planted some three decades ago. As video endoscopy was introduced, our endoscopy forefathers chose the color charge coupled device (CCD), while their Japanese counterparts used the black and white (B&W) CCD. The color CCD provided a lower resolution video, but was preferred because it used white light that was more pleasing to the eyes. The B&W CCD, on the other hand, used sequential red, green, and blue lights, which provides a superior imaging. However, it can appear to flicker and thus is less pleasing. With the lower quality endoscope imaging, western endoscopists have come to rely more on text and pathology to describe their findings, rather than on the detailed images. Thus, in the United States, the nonpolypoid precancers and early cancers were not appreciated. The techniques to enhance visualization of the nonpolypoid tumors were not prioritized, as few were found. Endoscopic mucosal resection techniques were not routine in the practice of endoscopy; there was no flat lesion to cut.

Since then, our CCD and endoscopy technology have significantly improved. With it came the recognition of the importance of the nonpolypoid tumors. But, generations of endoscopists were never taught the detection, diagnosis, or treatment techniques of the nonpolypoids. Thus, today, in the United States, we find ourselves with IBD practice guidelines that are outdated and endoscopy techniques that are largely ineffective. Of utmost concern, we lack the manuals and only have few teachers to disseminate the renewals. How are we then going to move forward?

The ubiquitous use of the electronic media may provide one avenue. We are indebted for the opportunity given by Dr Lightdale to prepare this issue, and to the contributing authors for their generosity to share knowledge. We are especially

Gastrointest Endoscopy Clin N Am 24 (2014) xv–xvi
http://dx.doi.org/10.1016/j.giec.2014.03.013
1052-5157/14/$ – see front matter © 2014 Published by Elsevier Inc.
giendo.theclinics.com

thankful to the Maxine and Jack Zarrow Family Foundation for their support to make this issue free online as a resource for all patients and health providers. Renaissance in endoscopic imaging in IBD can only begin when the patients demand, and the providers are able to deliver, the required care. Our sincere hope is that this (electronic) issue and atlas provide the first of the new guides in endoscopy for IBD. Thus, we can move forward and fulfill our promise—the Hippocratic Oath—to the fullest: "*I will apply, for the benefit of the sick, all measures [that] are required ....*" In the surveillance for colorectal neoplasms in patients with IBD, the art and science of the detection, diagnosis, and treatment of the nonpolypoid precancers and early cancers are required. We need to make them standard practice.

Tonya Kaltenbach, MD
Veterans Affairs Palo Alto
Stanford University School of Medicine
3801 Miranda Avenue, GI-111
Palo Alto, CA 94304, USA

Roy Soetikno, MD
Veterans Affairs Palo Alto
Stanford University School of Medicine
3801 Miranda Avenue, GI-111
Palo Alto, CA 94304, USA

E-mail addresses:
endoresection@me.com (T. Kaltenbach)
giendo@me.com (R. Soetikno)

Importance of Nonpolypoid (Flat and Depressed) Colorectal Neoplasms in Screening for CRC in Patients with IBD

CrossMark

Matthew D. Rutter, MBBS, MD, FRCP (London, Edinburgh)[a,b,*]

KEYWORDS

- Cancer • Dysplasia • Surveillance • Colonoscopy

KEY POINTS

- Patients with colitis have an increased risk of developing colorectal cancer (CRC), although the excess risk seems to be diminishing.
- Colonoscopic surveillance remains challenging because the cancer precursor (dysplasia) can have a varied endoscopic appearance.
- The vast majority of colitic dysplasia is endoscopically visible.
- The relative frequency of different dysplasia morphologies and true clinical significance of such lesions are difficult to determine from retrospective series, many of which were performed prior to the current era of endoscopic technique and imaging.

CANCER RISK

People with long-standing inflammatory bowel disease (IBD) colitis have a higher risk of developing CRC than the general population. The most reliable estimates of this risk come from population-based studies. The first such study, a large Swedish cohort of long-standing ulcerative colitis (UC), found a standardized incidence ratio (SIR) compared with the general population of 5.7 (95% CI, 4.6–7.0).[1] In more recent population-based studies of UC, the magnitude of risk seems smaller: an updated Swedish study found an SIR of 2.3 (95% CI, 2.0–2.6),[2] and one from Canada found an SIR of 2.75 (95% CI, 1.91–3.97).[3] Studies that have found no difference in CRC

[a] Department of Gastroenterology, University Hospital of North Tees, Hardwick, Stockton-on-Tees, Cleveland TS19 8PE, UK; [b] Durham University School of Medicine, Pharmacy and Health Queen's Campus, University Boulevard, Stockton-on-Tees, TS17 6BH, UK
* Department of Gastroenterology, University Hospital of North Tees, Hardwick, Stockton-on-Tees, Cleveland TS19 8PE, UK.
E-mail address: Matt.rutter@nth.nhs.uk

Gastrointest Endoscopy Clin N Am 24 (2014) 327–335
http://dx.doi.org/10.1016/j.giec.2014.03.002
1052-5157/14/$ – see front matter © 2014 Elsevier Inc. All rights reserved.

incidence or morbidity when comparing UC with the general population have in general been limited by selection bias[4] and retrospective study design.[5] A recent meta-analysis that summarizes the data from only population-based cohort studies found the risk of CRC 2.4-fold higher in UC compared with the general population.[6] Recent evidence suggests that the CRC risk in Crohn's colitis seems parallel to that in UC, for the same extent of colonic involvement. In Ekbom and colleagues' study,[7] patients with colonic Crohn had a relative risk (RR) of 5.6 (95% CI, 2.1–12.2) compared with the general population, in contrast to those with terminal ileal Crohn, who had a risk no different from the general population. Subsequent studies have corroborated these findings in Crohn's disease, reporting SIR of 2.1 (95% CI, 1.2–3.4)[2] and RR 2.64 (95% CI, 1.69–4.12).[3]

Various potential reasons for the apparent reduced risk of CRC over time have been postulated, including early study selection bias, differing means of determining colitis extent, timely colectomy, better disease (inflammation) control, a chemopreventive effect of aminosalicylate compounds, and the beneficial effect of surveillance programs.

Additional Risk Factors

Not all people with colitis have the same magnitude of CRC risk—several additional risk factors have been identified.

Extent of inflammation

Many studies (including a systematic review) have demonstrated that an increasing extent of mucosal inflammation correlates with increased CRC risk.[1,2,5,8,9] The measurement of disease extent has evolved over time: earliest studies used barium enemas, in contrast to more recent studies that have used either endoscopic (macroscopic) or histologic evidence. The original Swedish population-based study by Ekbom calculated a risk in UC for CRC of 1.7 for proctitis (nonsignificant), 2.8 for left-sided colitis, and 14.8 for pancolitis, compared with the general population.[1] Soderlund and colleagues'[2] updated study also indicated an increased risk, albeit of lower magnitude, with SIR 5.6 for pancolitis, 2.1 for Crohn's colitis, and 1.7 for proctitis—all statistically significantly higher than the general population. The underlying principle sustains—the more colonic mucosa involved, the greater the cancer risk to the patient.

Disease duration

A longer duration of colitis is associated with an increased risk of CRC. Early studies included in 2 meta-analyses indicated an exponentially increasing CRC risk after 10 years of UC,[10] with cumulative CRC risk of 2% at 10 years, 8% at 20 years, and 18% after 30 years of disease. More recent population-based studies have indicated, however, a much lower risk, with annual incidences as low as 0.06% to 0.20% and cumulative risk at 30 years as low as 2%.[4]

A Hungarian population-based study calculated a cumulative risk of 0.6% after 10 years, 5.4% after 20 years, and 7.5% after 30 years,[8] and, in the largest single-center study of colitis surveillance colonoscopy, the cumulative incidence of CRC by colitis duration showed a linear rather than exponential increase, from 2.5% at 20 years to 10.8% at 40 years of extensive UC.[11] CRC before 8 years of colitis was thought uncommon, although a recent Swedish study calculated that 17% to 22% of patients developed cancer before 8 to 10 years for extensive colitis and 15 to 20 years for left-sided disease.[12]

Severity of inflammation

IBD-CRC risk is thought to be promoted by inflammation. It is intuitive that more severe inflammation may confer a higher CRC risk, but early studies showed no clear association between colitic symptoms and CRC risk. There is poor correlation, however, between patients' symptoms and the severity of inflammation, and it was only when studies focused on severity of inflammation at a tissue level that the strong association became apparent. A British case-control study found a significant correlation between both colonoscopic (odds ratio [OR] 2.5, $P<.001$) and histologic (OR 5.1, $P<.001$) inflammation and neoplasia risk.[9] A second article on the same patient cohort found that macroscopically normal mucosa seemed to return the CRC risk to that of the general population.[13] A subsequent American cohort study then found a significant correlation between histologic inflammation and advanced neoplasia (hazard ratio 3.0; 95% CI, 1.4–6.3).[14]

Previous inflammation
Postinflammatory polyps (PIPs), which arise during healing after severe inflammation, have been associated with an increased CRC risk in 2 case-control studies, with ORs of 2.14 (95% CI, 1.24–3.70)[13] and 2.5 (95% CI, 1.4–4.6).[15] It is thought that this probably reflects the increased risk relating to previous severe inflammation rather than the PIPs having malignant potential per se.

Family history of CRC
As in noncolitic patients, a family history of CRC contributes to the risk of CRC in patients with colitis. Case-control and population-based studies show a 2- to 4-fold increase.[16] An American case-control study found family history of CRC an independent risk factor for UC-CRC (OR 3.7; 95% CI, 1.0–13.2).[15] A Swedish population-based study found that a family history of CRC was associated with a 2.5-fold increase in IBD-CRC (95% CI, 1.4–4.4). Where the first-degree relative was diagnosed with CRC before 50 years of age, the risk was even higher (RR 9.2; 95% CI, 3.7–23).[17]

Primary sclerosing cholangitis
Primary slerosing cholangitis (PSC) seems a particularly important independent risk factor for IBD-CRC. Although patients with PSC often have milder colonic inflammation, a meta-analysis of 11 studies concluded that patients who had both UC and PSC were at increased risk of CRC compared with patients with UC alone (OR 4.09; 95% CI, 2.89–5.76).[18] Cancers also often occur earlier in a patient's disease. Potential explanations include that such patients may have had subclinical inflammation for many years prior to colitis diagnosis, a deleterious effect of the altered bile salt pool, or possible shared genetic susceptibility of PSC and CRC.

Age at diagnosis
Young age at diagnosis may be a risk factor for IBD-CRC,[6] although data are inconsistent and may reflect other dependent factors (such as the potential for longer disease duration and more severe and extensive inflammation in younger age–onset patients).

Ekbom and colleagues'[1] population-based study found age at diagnosis an independent risk factor for CRC. Other studies have not confirmed this association. In Eaden and colleagues' meta-analysis,[10] a nonsignificant negative trend between younger age at onset and increased risk of CRC was seen in adult patients, although in children the cumulative risk of CRC was higher than the corresponding rates for adults. In a British 30-year study, patients who developed CRC had a higher median age of onset of disease than those not developing cancer.[11] Another study found a higher CRC risk in patients diagnosed with IBD above 30 to 40 years compared with those diagnosed before the age of 20.[19] A further study found that the time between onset of colitis and IBD-CRC was the same in young and old patients.[4] Although the lifetime risk and RR may be higher in those who develop colitis at a younger age, the absolute risk of developing CRC is higher in the elderly.[20]

Gender
Several studies have shown that the IBD-CRC risk is greater in men than in women.[6]

SURVEILLANCE
Evidence for Screening/Surveillance

Surveillance colonoscopy programs aim to reduce CRC mortality (by detecting cancer at an earlier stage with better prognosis) and where possible reduce CRC incidence (by detecting and resecting dysplasia), while preventing unnecessary surgery. The reduced CRC incidence seen in recent studies may be evidence that surveillance is effective, although there are other potential explanations (described previously). Three retrospective case-control studies have shown a correlation between the use of surveillance colonoscopy and reduced OR for CRC.[15,21,22] A Cochrane systematic review on the effectiveness of surveillance[23] was unable to demonstrate a benefit of surveillance programs for preventing CRC-related death in UC. Only 2 studies met their inclusion criteria, which was limited to cohort studies that included a control group. A more recent, larger cohort study showed improved survival from colonoscopic surveillance in IBD patients: 5-year CRC-related survival of patients on surveillance was 100% compared with 74% in the nonsurveillance group ($P = .042$).[24] In the surveillance group, 1 patient died as a consequence of CRC compared with 29 patients in the control group ($P = .047$) and more people with early tumor stage were found in the surveillance group ($P = .004$). All these studies could be subject to lead-time or selection bias; thus at present, unequivocal evidence of the benefit of colitis surveillance is lacking.

Because IBD-CRC tends to occur earlier in life than in the general population, benefit estimated in years of life saved may be much greater in colitis patients: mathematical models of life-years saved per case screened ranges from 14 to 60 months in UC patients compared with 1 to 4 months in general population screening.[23,25]

Appropriate Surveillance Strategy

Most societies recommend colonoscopic surveillance to address the increased CRC risk. No screening program, however, can be 100% effective. The detection and treatment of colorectal dysplasia in IBD remains problematic and, despite surveillance programs, patients still present with interval cancers. This may be because lesions are missed or are incompletely excised, because patients or clinicians do not comply with surveillance guidelines, or because aggressive de novo CRCs arise in between surveillance procedures.

The appropriate surveillance frequency is necessarily a pragmatic balance of cost (both financial and in terms of patient inconvenience and risk) and benefit. It is important to focus resources on those most at risk and most likely to benefit from the program. This is best achieved by using the established risk factors (detailed previously), and guidelines are increasingly using these for patient risk stratification.

Because duration of disease is a major risk factor for IBD-CRC, it is rational to commence surveillance colonoscopy when the risk starts to increase (ie, approximately 8–10 years after symptom onset).[10] The subsequent surveillance interval should take into account the risk for dysplasia development and the time it takes for dysplasia to progress to CRC. Unfortunately, the rate of dysplasia progression in IBD is not well established, although it undoubtedly varies between individuals. Therefore, intervals should be adjusted to individual patients according to their CRC risk factors.[26] Because CRCs have been detected within 2 years of surveillance colonoscopy, yearly colonoscopy seems appropriate for patients with high risk factors. The appropriate frequency of surveillance for other patients is less clear.

LESION CATEGORIZATION AND TERMINOLOGY
Dysplasia in Noncolitic Mucosa

Dysplastic lesions, polypoid or nonpolypoid, occurring in an area that has not been affected by inflammation can be assumed to be sporadic adenomas unrelated to the colitis and can be resected endoscopically.

Dysplasia Within Colitic Mucosa

Dysplasia within inflamed or previously inflamed mucosa is important because it may progress more rapidly than adenomas in noninflamed mucosa.[27] Thus, all such lesions should be removed promptly.

Endoscopically visible colitis-associated dysplasia—polypoid dysplasia

Most dysplasia is visible during colonoscopy,[28,29] and this proportion will continue to increase with ongoing improvements in endoscopic equipment and technique. Identification of dysplasia can be challenging, however, because it has a varied macroscopic appearance ranging from lesions that appear identical to sporadic adenomas to plaques, nodular mucosa, puckering of the mucosa, villiform mucosa, strictures, and broad-based masses with indistinct lateral margins. The relative incidence of each type of lesion has not been established in the modern era.

Raised dysplastic lesions within an area of current or previous inflammation have been termed dysplasia-associated lesions/masses (DALMs). Early studies showed high cancer incidences in such patients and until recently have been considered an indication for colectomy.[30] In many cases, the lesions were actually cancers, even though superficial mucosal biopsies did not demonstrate this endoscopically.

More recently, the term adenoma-like mass (ALM) has been used to describe dysplastic polyps within an area of colitis, which appear endoscopically similar to sporadic adenomas. ALMs are well-circumscribed, sessile, or pedunculated dysplastic polyps. Other terms used to describe these lesions have also been used, including adenoma-like DALMs and polypoid dysplasia.

Prompt, careful, and complete endoscopic resection of so-called ALMs (including negative biopsies taken from the normal-looking mucosa surrounding the polypectomy margins) carries a good prognosis even for invisible high-grade dysplasia (HGD), with overall rate of progression to cancer in a recent systematic review of only 2.4%.[31] If the lesion is not resectable, or is associated with dysplasia in the adjacent mucosa, then colectomy is appropriate due to the high risk of CRC.[28,30]

Unfortunately, there are no clear-cut histologic or immunohistochemical discriminators between DALMs, ALMs, and sporadic adenomas. Although some studies have shown that villous architecture, bottom-up as opposed to top-down crypt dysplasia, higher frequency of p53, lower frequency of KRAS mutations, and no surrounding dysplasia are more common in ALMs, none is specific enough for clinical use. Clinical management is thus best determined on the basis of endoscopic resectability. Because the use of the terms DALMs and ALMs has been inconsistent, leading to potential confusion and distortion of optimal management, they are best abandoned. Lesion morphology is best described using the Paris endoscopic classification.[32] A detailed endoscopic description of morphology, including whether the lesion is well circumscribed and whether there is background inflammation, is required.

Endoscopically visible colitis-associated dysplasia—nonpolypoid dysplasia

Flat dysplasia Many dysplastic lesions are polypoid (pedunculated or sessile and well-circumscribed). Just as in noncolitic patients, however, some lesions are minimally elevated (less than 2.5 mm in height, the width of closed biopsy forceps), completely flush with the mucosa, or even depressed in morphology. These are best described using Paris classification terminology: 0-IIa, 0-IIb, and 0-IIc lesions, respectively. To avoid terminology confusion, clinicians should only use the term, *flat*, in accordance with the Paris classification and should refrain from using the term, flat, to describe endoscopically unapparent (invisible) dysplasia.[32]

Nonpolypoid lesions can be more difficult to detect, particularly where background mucosa is inflamed or has postinflammatory changes, such as scarring or PIPs. Optimal detection is described in the article elsewhere in this issue. Once detected, however, many lesions may still be endoscopically resectable, after careful delineation of the lateral margin and inspection of the surrounding mucosa.

Strictures The finding of a stricture in patients with UC is always a concern. Clinicians should have a high index of suspicion that such strictures may harbor cancer. Even where this is not the case, there is a greatly increased risk of subsequent cancer development, with OR of 4.62 (95% CI, 1.03–20.8) in one case-control study.[13] Because biopsies may be falsely negative, surgery should be considered in such cases.

Endoscopically invisible colitis-associated dysplasia

Prior to the reclassification of colitis-associated dysplasia in 1983,[33] it was believed that dysplasia occurred as a field effect.[34] Based on an estimation that 33 biopsies were required to have a 90% chance of finding the highest degree of dysplasia present,[35] a policy of taking quadrantic random biopsies every 10 cm from the colorectum was recommended. This policy has been poorly adhered to, however, and is both costly and time consuming.[36] Because it is now recognized that the vast majority of colitic dysplasia is endoscopically visible, the recommendation to take multiple random biopsies of mucosa should be questioned. The true value of random biopsies has been demonstrated in the 10 prospective studies that have taken, per protocol, quadrantic random biopsies every 10 cm from the colorectum: on average 1 episode of dysplasia was detected for every 1505 random biopsies taken.[37] This time-consuming and expensive policy distracts endoscopists and should be abandoned in favor of careful mucosal inspection with targeted biopsies, aided by chromoendoscopy.

High-grade dysplasia Historical retrospective series and reviews indicate that when endoscopically invisible HGD is detected, there are high rates either of synchronous or metachronous cancer in 32% to 42% of patients. Thus, the general consensus among experts recommends colectomy for these patients.[38] Care must be taken with these historical and retrospective data, however, because it is likely that many of these lesions were not truly endoscopically invisible.

Low-grade dysplasia Where endoscopically invisible low-grade dysplasia (LGD) is detected, management is fraught with controversy because reported rates of progression to HGD or cancer vary from as low as 0% to greater than 50%.[39,40] Part of this variability relates to the challenge histopathologists have in a discriminating neoplastic from regenerative inflammatory changes, resulting in low interobserver agreement.[41] This is why guidelines recommend all colitis dysplasia is double-reported by an expert gastrointestinal pathologist. One recent meta-analysis revealed that the positive predictive value for progression from nonpolypoid LGD to HGD, dysplastic mass, or

CRC was 16%.[42] The significant variability in the underlying studies, however, must be stressed. Thus, the management decision (colectomy or surveillance) in the context of endoscopically invisible LGD remains challenging, should take into account other factors (such as other risk factors, comorbidity, age, solitary specimen, or synchronous/metachronous dysplasia), and should be made in conjunction with the patient and an experienced multidisciplinary clinical team.

Indefinite dysplasia Patients with biopsy specimens that show indefinite dysplasia have a risk of progression to HGD or CRC higher than in patients without dysplasia but lower than for LGD. Indefinite for dysplasia is not defined by specific criteria, and, as such, the diagnosis has high intra- and interobserver variability.

SUMMARY

Patients with IBD colitis have an increased risk of developing CRC compared with the general population. Colonoscopic surveillance remains challenging because the cancer precursor (dysplasia) can have a varied and subtle endoscopic appearance. Although historically the dysplasia was often considered endoscopically invisible, today with advanced endoscopic understanding, technique, and imaging, it is almost always visible. The frequency of different dysplasia morphologies and true clinical significance of such lesions are difficult to determine from retrospective series, many of which were performed prior to the current endoscopic era.

REFERENCES

1. Ekbom A, Helmick C, Zack M, et al. Ulcerative colitis and colorectal cancer. A population-based study. N Engl J Med 1990;323:1228–33.
2. Soderlund S, Brandt L, Lapidus A, et al. Decreasing time-trends of colorectal cancer in a large cohort of patients with inflammatory bowel disease. Gastroenterology 2009;136:1561–7.
3. Bernstein CN, Blanchard JF, Kliewer E, et al. Cancer risk in patients with inflammatory bowel disease: a population-based study. Cancer 2001;91:854–62.
4. Winther KV, Jess T, Langholz E, et al. Long-term risk of cancer in ulcerative colitis: a population-based cohort study from Copenhagen County. Clin Gastroenterol Hepatol 2004;2:1088–95.
5. Jess T, Loftus EV Jr, Velayos FS, et al. Risk of intestinal cancer in inflammatory bowel disease: a population-based study from olmsted county, Minnesota. Gastroenterology 2006;130:1039–46.
6. Jess T, Rungoe C, Peyrin-Biroulet L. Risk of colorectal cancer in patients with ulcerative colitis: a meta-analysis of population-based cohort studies. Clin Gastroenterol Hepatol 2012;10(6):639–45.
7. Ekbom A, Helmick C, Zack M, et al. Increased risk of large-bowel cancer in Crohn's disease with colonic involvement. Lancet 1990;336:357–9.
8. Lakatos L, Mester G, Erdelyi Z, et al. Risk factors for ulcerative colitis-associated colorectal cancer in a Hungarian cohort of patients with ulcerative colitis: results of a population-based study. Inflamm Bowel Dis 2006;12:205–11.
9. Rutter M, Saunders B, Wilkinson K, et al. Severity of inflammation is a risk factor for colorectal neoplasia in ulcerative colitis. Gastroenterology 2004;126:451–9.
10. Eaden JA, Abrams KR, Mayberry JF. The risk of colorectal cancer in ulcerative colitis: a meta-analysis. Gut 2001;48:526–35.

11. Rutter MD, Saunders BP, Wilkinson KH, et al. Thirty-year analysis of a colono-scopic surveillance program for neoplasia in ulcerative colitis. Gastroenterology 2006;130:1030–8.

12. Lutgens MW, Vleggaar FP, Schipper ME, et al. High frequency of early colorectal cancer in inflammatory bowel disease. Gut 2008;57(9):1246–51.

13. Rutter MD, Saunders BP, Wilkinson KH, et al. Cancer surveillance in longstanding ulcerative colitis: endoscopic appearances help predict cancer risk. Gut 2004; 53:1813–6.

14. Gupta RB, Harpaz N, Itzkowitz S, et al. Histologic inflammation is a risk factor for progression to colorectal neoplasia in ulcerative colitis: a cohort study. Gastroen-terology 2007;133:1099–105.

15. Velayos FS, Loftus EV Jr, Jess T, et al. Predictive and protective factors associ-ated with colorectal cancer in ulcerative colitis: a case-control study. Gastroenter-ology 2006;130:1941–9.

16. Nuako KW, Ahlquist DA, Mahoney DW, et al. Familial predisposition for colorectal cancer in chronic ulcerative colitis: a case-control study. Gastroenterology 1998; 115:1079–83.

17. Askling J, Dickman PW, Karlen P, et al. Family history as a risk factor for colorectal cancer in inflammatory bowel disease. Gastroenterology 2001;120:1356–62.

18. Soetikno RM, Lin OS, Heidenreich PA, et al. Increased risk of colorectal neoplasia in patients with primary sclerosing cholangitis and ulcerative colitis: a meta-anal-ysis. Gastrointest Endosc 2002;56:48–54.

19. Greenstein AJ, Sachar DB, Smith H, et al. Cancer in universal and left-sided ulcerative colitis: factors determining risk. Gastroenterology 1979;77:290–4.

20. Beaugerie L, Svrcek M, Seksik P, et al. Risk of colorectal high-grade dysplasia and cancer in a prospective observational cohort of patients with inflammatory bowel disease. Gastroenterology 2013;145:166–75.e8.

21. Karlen P, Kornfeld D, Brostrom O, et al. Is colonoscopic surveillance reducing colorectal cancer mortality in ulcerative colitis? A population based case control study. Gut 1998;42:711–4.

22. Eaden J, Abrams K, Ekbom A, et al. Colorectal cancer prevention in ulcerative colitis: a case-control study. Aliment Pharmacol Ther 2000;14:145–53.

23. Collins PD, Mpofu C, Watson AJ, et al. Strategies for detecting colon cancer and/ or dysplasia in patients with inflammatory bowel disease. Cochrane Database Syst Rev 2006;(2):CD000279.

24. Lutgens MW, Oldenburg B, Siersema PD, et al. Colonoscopic surveillance im-proves survival after colorectal cancer diagnosis in inflammatory bowel disease. Br J Cancer 2009;101:1671–5.

25. Provenzale D, Wong JB, Onken JE, et al. Performing a cost-effectiveness anal-ysis: surveillance of patients with ulcerative colitis. Am J Gastroenterol 1998;93: 872–80.

26. Cairns SR, Scholefield JH, Steele RJ, et al. Guidelines for colorectal cancer screening and surveillance in moderate and high risk groups (update from 2002). Gut 2010;59:666–89.

27. Vieth M, Behrens H, Stolte M. Sporadic adenoma in ulcerative colitis: endoscopic resection is an adequate treatment. Gut 2006;55:1151–5.

28. Rutter MD, Saunders BP, Wilkinson KH, et al. Most dysplasia in ulcerative colitis is visible at colonoscopy. Gastrointest Endosc 2004;60:334–9.

29. Rubin DT, Rothe JA, Hetzel JT, et al. Are dysplasia and colorectal cancer endo-scopically visible in patients with ulcerative colitis? Gastrointest Endosc 2007;65: 998–1004.

30. Blackstone MO, Riddell RH, Rogers BH, et al. Dysplasia-associated lesion or mass (DALM) detected by colonoscopy in long-standing ulcerative colitis: an indication for colectomy. Gastroenterology 1981;80:366–74.
31. Wanders LW, Dekker E, Pullens B, et al. Cancer risk after resection of polypoid dysplasia in patients with longstanding ulcerative colitis: a meta-analysis. Clin Gastroenterol Hepatol 2014;12(5):756–64.
32. The Paris endoscopic classification of superficial neoplastic lesions: esophagus, stomach, and colon: November 30 to December 1, 2002. Gastrointest Endosc 2003;58:S3–43.
33. Riddell RH, Goldman H, Ransohoff DF, et al. Dysplasia in inflammatory bowel disease: standardized classification with provisional clinical applications. Hum Pathol 1983;14:931–68.
34. Morson BC, Pang LS. Rectal biopsy as an aid to cancer control in ulcerative colitis. Gut 1967;8:423–34.
35. Rubin CE, Haggitt RC, Burmer GC, et al. DNA aneuploidy in colonic biopsies predicts future development of dysplasia in ulcerative colitis. Gastroenterology 1992; 103:1611–20.
36. Eaden JA, Ward BA, Mayberry JF. How gastroenterologists screen for colonic cancer in ulcerative colitis: an analysis of performance [see comments]. Gastrointest Endosc 2000;51:123–8.
37. Rutter MD, Riddell RH. Colorectal dysplasia in inflammatory bowel disease: a clinicopathological perspective. Clin Gastroenterol Hepatol 2014;12(3):359–67.
38. Bernstein CN, Shanahan F, Weinstein WM. Are we telling patients the truth about surveillance colonoscopy in ulcerative colitis? [see comments] [review]. Lancet 1994;343:71–4.
39. Connell WR, Lennard-Jones JE, Williams CB, et al. Factors affecting the outcome of endoscopic surveillance for cancer in ulcerative colitis [see comments]. Gastroenterology 1994;107:934–44.
40. Jess T, Loftus EV Jr, Velayos FS, et al. Incidence and prognosis of colorectal dysplasia in inflammatory bowel disease: a population-based study from Olmsted County, Minnesota. Inflamm Bowel Dis 2006;12:669–76.
41. Dixon MF, Brown LJ, Gilmour HM, et al. Observer variation in the assessment of dysplasia in ulcerative colitis. Histopathology 1988;13:385–97.
42. Thomas T, Abrams KA, Robinson RJ, et al. Meta-analysis: cancer risk of low-grade dysplasia in chronic ulcerative colitis. Aliment Pharmacol Ther 2007;25: 657–68.

Interval Colorectal Cancers in Inflammatory Bowel Disease: The Grim Statistics and True Stories

Silvia Sanduleanu, MD, PhD[a],*,
Matthew D. Rutter, MBBS, MD, FRCP (London, Edinburgh)[b,c]

KEYWORDS

- Colorectal cancer • Interval colorectal cancer • Inflammatory bowel disease
- Ulcerative colitis • Crohn's disease • Surveillance • Colonoscopy

KEY POINTS

- Interval colorectal cancers (CRCs) may account for approximately half of all CRCs identified during IBD surveillance, which highlights the need for improvements.
- The cause of interval CRCs is multifactorial, with procedural factors likely to play an important role.
- Molecular events promoted by inflamed mucosa may augment the cancer risk and perhaps explain some interval CRCs.

The past decade has witnessed considerable progress in the management of inflammatory bowel disease (IBD), including improvements in the quality and effectiveness of colonoscopic surveillance.[1-3] Patients with ulcerative colitis (UC) or Crohn's colitis have a greater risk of colorectal cancers (CRC), which may develop earlier and progress more rapidly than sporadic CRCs. Although most societies now endorse intensive colonoscopic surveillance to reduce the CRC risk,[4-6] the efficacy of this strategy remains controversial. Several recent studies have cast doubt about the limited effectiveness of colonoscopy at reducing the incidence of sporadic CRC in the general population, especially in the proximal part of the colon,[7,8] resulting in the occurrence of interval CRCs. Little is known, however, about the magnitude of this problem in patients with IBD and the most common explanations. Similar to the sporadic interval CRCs, two factors contribute to interval CRCs in IBD: clinician-dependent factors, such as missed, incompletely resected lesions or suboptimal surveillance; and

[a] Division of Gastroenterology and Hepatology, Department of Internal Medicine, GROW, School for Oncology and Developmental Biology, Maastricht University Medical Center, Postbox 5800, 6202 AZ, Maastricht, The Netherlands; [b] Department of Gastroenterology, University Hospital of North Tees, Hardwick, Stockton-on-Tees, Cleveland, TS19 8PE, UK; [c] Durham University School of Medicine, Pharmacy and Health Queen's Campus, University Boulevard, Stockton-on-Tees, Cleveland, TS17 6BH, UK
* Corresponding author.
E-mail address: s.sanduleanu@mumc.nl

Gastrointest Endoscopy Clin N Am 24 (2014) 337–348
http://dx.doi.org/10.1016/j.giec.2014.03.001
1052-5157/14/$ – see front matter © 2014 Elsevier Inc. All rights reserved.

molecular features of the inflamed mucosa underlying the development of cancer. The endoscopic knowledge, equipment, and techniques have evolved in recent years, contributing to a paradigm shift in the diagnosis and endoscopic resection of CRC precursors. The nonpolypoid (flat or depressed) colorectal neoplasms (NP-CRNs) play a significant role in the genesis of interval CRCs.[9] Such subtle-appearing lesions are indeed more likely missed or incompletely resected endoscopically than their polypoid counterparts, and a subgroup of them harbor an aggressive biologic behavior.

This article provides insight into the magnitude and most common factors underlying the cause of interval CRCs during surveillance for IBD. Milestones of the literature regarding CRC risk in patients with IBD are reviewed. Specifically examined to the occurrence of interval CRCs are the contribution of missed, incompletely resected lesions; the adherence to surveillance; and distinct biologic features of the inflamed mucosa. Key principles are presented for ensuring the quality of IBD surveillance practice.

INCIDENCE OF CRC AND INTERVAL CRC

A casual glance at the overall incidence of CRC in patients with IBD reveals discrepant outcomes, with a few studies showing similar CRC rates in patients with IBD versus the general population,[10,11] whereas others show greater rates.[12–14] In a nationwide cohort of close to 50,000 Danish patients with IBD who were followed over three decades (1979–2008), CRC was identified in 338 (0.71%) cases (268 in patients with UC and 70 in patients with Crohn's disease).[10] The overall CRC risk among patients with UC in this study was similar to that of the general population (relative risk, 1.07; 95% confidence interval, 0.95–1.21). In contrast, a North American study[15] conducted from 1998 through 2010 found that the incidence of CRC in patients with Crohn's disease or UC was 60% higher than in the general population.

The Danish study found a marked decline in the overall relative risk of CRC among patients with UC over the past decades, from 1.34 (95% confidence interval, 1.13–1.58) in 1979 to 1988 to 0.57 (95% confidence interval, 0.41–0.80) in 1999 to 2008,[10] possibly reflecting refinements in the anti-inflammatory arsenal (ie, immunosuppressive therapy, biologicals), but perhaps also caused by a gradual adoption of CRC screening and surveillance. Conversely, the North American study[15] found a fairly stable CRC rate in patients with IBD over time. Controversies surrounding the time-trends in CRC risk are not surprising, and likely reflect the cumulative effect of several factors, such as advancements in endoscope technology, a greater awareness, and improvements in the quality of colonoscopic performance.

As a common denominator, such epidemiologic studies lack relevant information about the disease duration, degree and extent of inflammation, presence of risk factors (ie, primary sclerosing cholangitis, personal or family history of CRC), and patients' compliance with the recommended follow-up. Although clinical studies provide such details, most have focused on the optimal frequency of surveillance, paying less attention to the quality of examination. A systematic characterization of the lesions phenotype, in particular the location, size, shape, and histology, is often lacking.

Very few data are available about the occurrence of interval cancers during surveillance for IBD. The first paper dates back to 1982.[16] In this surgical review of 676 patients with UC undergoing long-term follow-up, a total of 35 CRCs were identified. Twelve of these were diagnosed because of symptoms, 10 as incidental findings at proctocolectomy, and 13 CRCs were diagnosed during the follow-up at least 1 year after the initial UC diagnosis. This latter subgroup was referred to as "interval CRCs." In a St Mark's study reviewing the UC surveillance program over approximately three decades, a total of 74 patients (12.3% of the total population) developed neoplasms, including 30 CRCs.[17] The authors defined interval CRCs as "cancers presenting after a negative index-colonoscopy or advanced (Dukes' C/disseminated) cancers detected at surveillance." During a median follow-up of 1.5 years, nine patients were identified with Dukes' C cancers and four patients with disseminated cancers (4 of these 13 cases were diagnosed within 12 months). In three cases, CRC was diagnosed at colonoscopy because of symptoms; one of these was attributable to noncompliance. Of note, more than half (16 out of the 30) of the CRCs identified with this program were interval cancers, raising concerns about the effectiveness of colonoscopic cancer prevention. A statistically significant reduction in CRC rates over time was observed in this study ($r = -0.40$; $P = .04$), especially in the proximal colon.

From these data, we can conclude that there is sparse understanding of the magnitude and clinical significance of interval CRCs in patients with IBD. Indeed, a wide variation exists with regard to the terminology used in endoscopy and pathology diagnostic protocols across countries, IBD centers, and studies.

Standardization of the nomenclature and clinical protocols, and uniformity in reporting on interval CRCs during IBD surveillance, would help to define quality targets. As a first step, a universal terminology is required for dysplasia and interval cancers. Previously used terms, such as flat dysplasia or dysplasia associated lesion or mass, need to be revisited. A rigorous description of the endoscopic shape and histologic features of the detected lesions is required, using international classifications (ie, Paris-Japanese endoscopic classifications[18,19] and the World Health Organization histopathologic classifications[20,21]). Interval cancers should be considered those invasive cancers diagnosed after a negative screening examination, but before the next recommended follow-up colonoscopy, as endorsed by the current international IBD surveillance guidelines.

POTENTIAL ETIOLOGIC FACTORS OF INTERVAL CRCS

Similarly to sporadic CRCs, most interval CRCs in IBD probably can be explained by clinician-dependent factors, such as missed, incompletely resected lesions or deviation from surveillance protocols. The understanding of the underpinnings of such interval CRCs is of importance because it may permit identification of modifiable factors, for example gaps in knowledge and training on the recognition of nonpolypoid neoplasms and their endoscopic resection. In this case, tailored educational programs would improve the awareness and help to shape practical skills, to ultimately safeguard the quality of colonoscopy. Furthermore, it is important to understand whether certain molecular features of the inflamed mucosa could augment the risk of cancer progression. Such information may help to develop personalized (ie, molecular-based) surveillance strategies.

Missed Lesions

Two recent studies exploring the cause of sporadic interval CRCs in the general population found missed lesions represent by far the most important contributor (>50% of all interval CRCs).[22,23] Undoubtedly, missed lesions are likely to account for a significant proportion of interval CRCs in IBD, although a thorough analysis using structured algorithms[24] has not yet been performed. A recent population-based analysis by Wang and colleagues,[25] using SEER cancer registry data from 55,008 older patients with CRC, found rates of early/missed CRCs were three-fold greater in IBD than in patients without IBD (15.1% for Crohn's disease, 15.8% for UC vs 5.8% for patients without IBD; $P<.001$). Early/missed CRCs were defined as CRCs identified within 6 to 36 months after a colonoscopic examination that did not detect cancer. This study was based on administrative data, and therefore lacked detail about the completeness of colonoscopy, bowel preparation, extent of colitis, characteristics of mucosal lesions identified at the baseline examination, and resection outcomes. Such observations underscore the importance of meticulous inspection of the entire colonic mucosa, which should be ideally clean and free of inflammation, and the need for formal training of the endoscopist in the recognition of IBD neoplasms. Presence of active or chronic background inflammation and the diversity in endoscopic appearance of dysplasia by IBD may, however, increase the complexity of diagnosis. **Fig. 1** illustrates a lateral spreading tumor of granular subtype, which could have been missed at a previous examination.

A substantial number of studies demonstrated that indigo carmine– or methylene blue–guided chromoendoscopy (CE) improves the diagnostic yield of dysplasia and

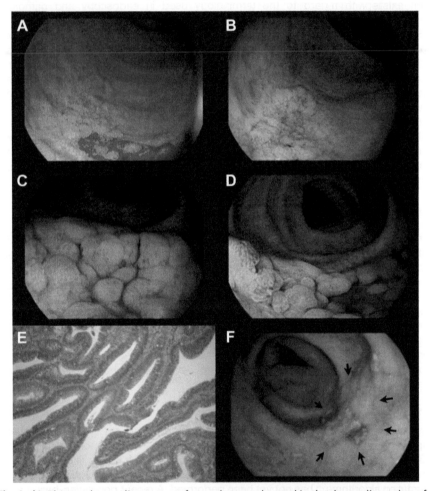

Fig. 1. (*A–D*) Lateral spreading tumor of granular type, located in the descending colon of a patient with a Crohn's pancolitis. (*E*) Histopathology revealed low-grade dysplasia (Hematoxylin and eosin, original magnification ×20). (*F*) Colonoscopic examination 8 months earlier showed Mayo 2 inflammation only at the same anatomic site (*arrows*), suggesting this lesion could have been missed.

invasive CRC during IBD surveillance. This is not surprising, because a significant proportion[26–28] of dysplastic lesions in patients with IBD appear to have a flat appearance, as illustrated in **Table 1**. Pancolonic CE delineates the borders and permits a detailed analysis of the epithelial surface, thus facilitating the diagnosis of subtle lesions and their endoscopic resection. A few meta-analyses now demonstrate CE with targeted biopsies is superior to white-light colonoscopy with random biopsies in the detection of dysplasia and invasive CRCs.[29–31] CE yielded a 7% increase in the detection of any dysplasia.[31] Compared with white-light colonoscopy with random biopsies, the likelihood to detect any dysplasia with CE and targeted biopsies was 8.9-fold greater, and 5.2-fold greater for detecting nonpolypoid dysplasia. In a Mainz study of 165 patients with long-standing UC who were randomized to undergo standard colonoscopy using white light versus CE (0.1% methylene blue), significantly more intraepithelial neoplasms were detected in the CE group (32 vs 10; $P = .003$). CE detected more intraepithelial neoplasms in "flat mucosa" than white-light endoscopy (24 vs 4; $P = .0007$), and more invasive cancers (3 vs 1).[26]

In these studies, colonoscopies were performed by dedicated colonoscopists with expertise in multimodal imaging, and under controlled circumstances (ie, clinical trials), and may preclude generalizability. Recognition of the nonpolypoid dysplasia in a real-world environment remains challenging and requires additional training. In a study conducted at Maastricht University Medical Center, where the endoscopists have been trained on the recognition of nonpolypoid neoplasms,[32] the overall detection rate of sporadic NP-CRNs (defined as lesions of which the height was less than half of the diameter) was 5.7% (diagnostic subgroup, 4.7%; screening subgroup, 4.5%; surveillance subgroup, 15.6%).[33] The learning-curve in the detection of NP-CRNs is, however, tedious, with at least 600 colonoscopies being required to achieve a detection rate of at least 4.5%.[34]

It is highly likely that missed lesions have a major contribution to the development of interval CRCs in patients with IBD, although this needs further investigation. The current data highlight the importance of vigilant inspection and a thorough phenotyping of lesions identified at colonoscopy, including subtle erosions, shallow ulcerations, and their relationship with inflammation or strictures. Such exquisite detail may improve the understanding of the link between inflammation, the occurrence of dysplasia, and interval CRCs. High-quality videos/photodocumentation obtained in a standardized fashion facilitates this process. Challenging cases should be performed by expert endoscopists.

Incompletely Resected Lesions

Endoscopic resection of neoplasms in the context of colitis is clearly fraught with difficulties because of the presence of inflammation and scarring. Such conditions challenge the accurate detection, clear demarcation, and lifting of the lesions. Studies examining the diagnostic yield of CE during surveillance for IBD provided, however, limited information about the effectiveness of the endoscopic resection, which requires further investigation. In a long-term follow-up evaluation, Odze and colleagues[35] compared the outcome after polypectomy among three subgroups: (1) patients with UC with adenoma-like dysplastic lesions, (2) patients with UC with sporadic adenomas, and (3) a non-UC sporadic adenoma subgroup. Prevalence of polyp formation on follow-up, albeit high in this study, did not significantly differ across subgroups (62.5%, 50%, and 49%, respectively) indicating IBD-associated dysplasia may be effectively treated endoscopically. Indeed, over the past few years, endoscopic mucosal resection and endoscopic submucosal dissection resection techniques proved to be increasingly safe and effective in the Western practice.[36–38] A study

Table 1
Detection of flat dysplastic lesions in patients undergoing surveillance for IBD

Study, Author, Year	Design	Endoscopist Experience	Number of Patients	Dye	Number of Patients with IEN	Flat Dysplastic Lesions (Numbers)	Invasive CRCs (Numbers)
Kiesslich et al,[26] 2003	Randomized 1:1, CE vs standard WLE	Several experienced endoscopists	165	MB 0.1%	CE group: 32 IENs in 13 pts WLE group: 10 IENs in 6 pts	CE group: 24 WLE group: 4 (P = .0007)	CE group: 3 invasive CRC WLE group: 1 invasive CRC
Matsumoto et al,[27] 2003	Prospective cohort CE	Single experienced endoscopist	57	IC 0.2%	12 pts with 117 IENs	27	4 HGD/invasive CRCs
Rutter et al,[28] 2004	Prospective cohort back-to-back WLE→CE	Single experienced endoscopist	100	IC 0.1%	CE group: 9 pts WLE group: 2 pts	CE group: 75 "flat topped elevated" WLE group: 0	None
Kiesslich et al, 2007	Randomized 1:1 CE (N = 80) vs WLE (N = 73)	Several experienced endoscopists	153	MB 0.1%	CE group: 19 in 11 pts CC group: 4 in 4 pts	CE group: 16 CC group: 2	None
Hlavaty et al, 2011	Tandem colonoscopies	Several experienced endoscopists	30	IC 0.4%	WLE: 2 CE: 4	2	None
Günther et al, 2011	Randomized Group 1: random biopsies; Group 2 CE + biopsies; Group 3 CE + confocal endomicroscopy	Two experienced endoscopists	150	IC 0.1%	Group 1: no IEN Group 2: 2 pts Group 3: 4 pts	Group I (0) Group II (18) Group III (10)	1 (Group 3)

Abbreviations: CC, conventional colonoscopy; HGD, high-grade dysplasia; IC, indigo carmine; MB, methylene blue; WLE, white-light endoscopy.

examining the effectiveness of endoscopic resection of NP-CRNs found that 93% of those larger than 10 mm were successfully resected.[36] Residual neoplasia was identified in 10% of cases on the first follow-up examination, although complete resection was obtained in all cases after one to three follow-up examinations. Likewise, Buchner and colleagues[37] found that large sessile and NP-CRNs could be managed endoscopically in 91% of cases, with a perforation rate of 0.4% and a bleeding rate of 11%. Because 9%[23] to 50%[38] of the sporadic interval CRCs are thought to be caused by an ineffective polyp resection, the precise contribution of this factor to the genesis of interval CRCs in patients with IBD needs further elucidation.

Adherence to Colonoscopic Surveillance

Adherence to colonoscopic surveillance guidelines is indeed vital, but seems to be often problematic.[39–42] There are several caveats to keep in mind, foremost of which is the patient's understanding of the cancer risk.[43,44] Disease flares and presence of comorbidity may further reduce the compliance to surveillance. Because the presence of disease activity challenges the endoscopic and histologic appreciation of dysplasia, colonoscopic surveillance should be ideally performed in the quiescent phase. However, surveillance should not be delayed too long, because those with more active disease carry a greater risk of developing CRC. With regard to bowel preparation, a low-residue diet the days before the procedure in conjunction with split-dose polyethylene glycol solutions is often sufficient for adequate cleansing, without inducing inflammation.

Biologic Features

The precise biologic events underlying chronic inflammation and leading to a faster progression to CRC are presently unknown and need further exploration. A subset of dysplastic lesions identified in patients with IBD harbor a villous phenotype, as illustrated in **Fig. 2**. Such macroscopic features have been suggested to represent a red flag for the presence of invasive CRC, especially of colloid subtype.[45] Other CRCs harbor signet ring cells, features associated with a more aggressive biologic behavior. **Fig. 3** illustrates a small signet ring cell carcinoma that displayed clear signs of local invasion. Approximately 6% of the cancers in patients with IBD are small flat invasive CRCs, without adjacent adenomatous tissue,[30] suggesting that progression to CRC may involve a pathway different from the classic adenoma-carcinoma sequence.

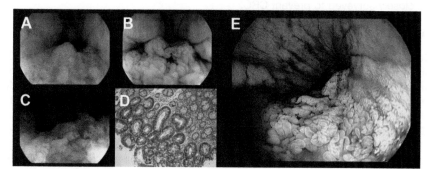

Fig. 2. (*A–C*) Lateral spreading tumor of the rectum in a patient with distal ulcerative colitis. Examination using high-definition endoscopy in conjunction with chromoendoscopy clearly showed a villous appearance. (*D*) Histopathology revealed low-grade dysplasia (Hematoxylin and eosin, original magnification ×20). (*E*) Fuller view of lesion with indigo carmine chromoendoscopy.

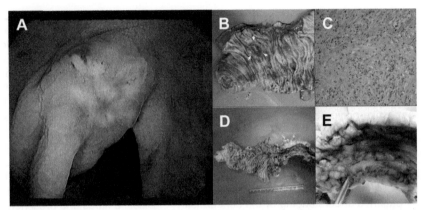

Fig. 3. (*A*) A 10-mm sized, Paris type IIa+IIc lesion, with a central ulceration that has been identified at the hepatic flexure of a patient with Crohn's colitis. (*B*) Examination of the surgical specimen showed the small cancer (*arrows*). (*C*) Histopathology revealed a poorly differentiated signet ring cell adenocarcinoma, with signs of lymphangioinvasion. The lesion was located near a stricture (Hematoxylin and eosin, original magnification ×30) (*D*, *E*) and staged pT3N1Mx.

The newly described serrated neoplastic pathway may also explain a subset of interval CRCs in patients with IBD.[46] Interestingly, a recent study by Voorham and colleagues[47] found that sporadic nonpolypoid neoplasms are likely to herald 5q loss, and less likely MSI and APC mutations, features resembling the carcinogenesis process in inflammatory conditions, such as IBD.

In summary, clinician-dependent factors and biologic factors intermingle in the genesis of interval CRCs by IBD. It is important to understand whether presence of NP (flat or depressed)-CRNs in patients with IBD signifies a diagnostic and therapeutic challenge alone. The most effective filter of missed or incompletely resected lesions would then be training for improving the education and endoscopic skills. Clinical decisional algorithms, including the characterization of shape, epithelial surface of lesions, and their relation with inflammation,[31] have the potential to steer the diagnostic and therapeutic process and optimize outcomes. If a subset of the NP-CRNs contains molecular features associated with a greater risk of CRC, such patients need to be identified and closely surveyed to prevent CRC.

CONCLUDING REMARKS

Interval CRCs may account for approximately 50% of the CRCs identified during IBD surveillance, favoring the idea that clinical consent should include information about cancer risk. Improvements in the quality of colonoscopic examinations are vital for minimizing the CRC risk of patients with IBD. **Box 1** summarizes basic concepts for achieving that goal. Standardization of clinical protocols is required, including the use of high-definition and high-resolution colonoscopes coupled with the application of pancolonic CE with targeted biopsies. Surveillance colonoscopy using white light with random biopsies should be abandoned. Formal training in recognition of NP-CRNs and proficiency in endoscopic resection techniques should be compulsory for providers who perform surveillance in patients with IBD. Comprehensive colonoscopy and pathology data reporting using a standardized nomenclature and interpretation of findings using tailored algorithms may ultimately shed light on the cause of interval CRCs and the required improvements.

Box 1
Principles for quality colonoscopy during surveillance for IBD: The Six Ts

- Timing

  Ideally, surveillance should be performed in the quiescent phase.

- Tolerance

  Tolerance of bowel preparation is key for adequate cleansing; a low-residue diet can be added to standard split-dose bowel preparations.

- Technology

  High-definition/high-resolution colonoscopes should be used.

- Technique

  Pancolonic chromoendoscopy with targeted biopsies should be considered the standard of care.

- Training

  The IBD specialist and pathologist needs to be formally trained on detection, classification, and diagnosis of nonpolypoid (flat or depressed) colorectal neoplasms.

- Traits

  A thorough registration of patient and lesion characteristics may help identify the most likely cause:

  o Patient with IBD: duration and extent of disease, presence of primary sclerosing cholangitis, family history of CRC, personal history of colorectal polyps (including postinflammatory polyps), history of medication, compliance and response to therapy

  o Lesions at baseline examination: location, size, shape, histology, and the relationship with inflammation and strictures

  o Interval CRCs: recommended surveillance intervals, time to CRC diagnosis, location of tumor, histology, and tumor stage

---

REFERENCES

1. Mowat C, Cole A, Windsor A, et al. Guidelines for the management of inflammatory bowel disease in adults. Gut 2011;60(5):571–607.
2. Rutter MD, Riddell RH. Colorectal dysplasia in inflammatory bowel disease: a clinicopathologic perspective. Clin Gastroenterol Hepatol 2014;12(3): 359–67.
3. Murthy SK, Kiesslich R. Evolving endoscopic strategies for detection and treatment of neoplastic lesions in inflammatory bowel disease. Gastrointest Endosc 2013;77(3):351–9.
4. Cairns SR, Scholefield JH, Steele RJ, et al. Guidelines for colorectal cancer screening and surveillance in moderate and high-risk groups (update from 2002). Gut 2010;59(5):666–89.
5. Farraye FA, Odze RD, Eaden J, et al. AGA technical review on the diagnosis and management of colorectal neoplasia in inflammatory bowel disease. Gastroenterology 2010;138(2):746–74.
6. Kornbluth A, Sachar DB, Practice Parameters Committee of the American College of Gastroenterology. Ulcerative colitis practice guidelines in adults (update): American College of Gastroenterology, Practice parameters Committee. Am J Gastroenterol 2004;99(7):1371–85.

7. Lakoff J, Paszat LF, Saskin R, et al. Risk of developing proximal versus distal colorectal cancer after a negative colonoscopy: a population-based study. Clin Gastroenterol Hepatol 2008;10:1117–21.

8. Brenner H, Chang-Claude J, Seiler CM, et al. Protection from colorectal cancer after colonoscopy: a population-based, case-control study. Ann Intern Med 2011;154(1):22–30.

9. Sanduleanu S, Masclee AM, Meijer GA. Interval cancers after colonoscopy: insights and recommendations. Nat Rev Gastroenterol Hepatol 2012;9(9):550–4.

10. Jess T, Simonsen J, Jørgensen KT, et al. Decreasing risk of colorectal cancer in patients with inflammatory bowel disease over 30 years. Gastroenterology 2012; 143(2):375–81.

11. Kappelman MD, Farkas DK, Long MD, et al. Risk of cancer in patients with inflammatory bowel diseases: a nationwide population-based cohort study with 30 years of follow-up evaluation. Clin Gastroenterol Hepatol 2014;12(2): 265–73.e1.

12. Eaden JA, Abrams KR, Mayberry JF. The risk of colorectal cancer in ulcerative colitis: a meta-analysis. Gut 2001;48(4):526–35.

13. Ekbom A, Helmick C, Zack M, et al. Ulcerative colitis and colorectal cancer. A population-based study. N Engl J Med 1990;323(18):1228–33.

14. Mellemkjaer L, Olsen JH, Frisch M, et al. Cancer in patients with ulcerative colitis. Int J Cancer 1995;60(3):330–3.

15. Herrinton LJ, Liu L, Levin TR, et al. Incidence and mortality of colorectal adenocarcinomas in persons with inflammatory bowel disease from 1998 to 2010. Gastroenterology 2012;143(2):382–9.

16. Prior P, Gyde SN, Macartney JC, et al. Cancer morbidity in ulcerative colitis. Gut 1982;23(6):490–7.

17. Rutter MD, Saunders BP, Wilkinson KH, et al. Thirty-year analysis of a colonoscopic surveillance program for neoplasia in ulcerative colitis. Gastroenterology 2006;130(4):1030–8.

18. Kudo S, Lambert R, Allen JI, et al. Nonpolypoid neoplastic lesions of the colorectal mucosa. Gastrointest Endosc 2008;68(Suppl 4):S3–47.

19. Soetikno R, Friedland S, Kaltenbach T, et al. Nonpolypoid (flat and depressed) colorectal neoplasms. Gastroenterology 2006;130:566–76.

20. Hamilton S, Aaltonen LA. WHO classification of tumours. Pathology and genetics: tumours of the digestive system. Lyon (France): IARC; 2000.

21. Bosman FT, Carneiro F, Hruban RH, et al. WHO classification of tumours. Pathology and genetics. Tumours of the digestive system. 4th edition. Berlin: Springer-Verlag; 2010.

22. Robertson DJ, Lieberman DA, Winawer SJ, et al. Colorectal cancers soon after colonoscopy: a pooled multicohort analysis. Gut 2013. [Epub ahead of print].

23. Le Clercq CM, Bouwens MW, Rondagh EJ, et al. Postcolonoscopy colorectal cancers are preventable: a population-based study. Gut 2013. [Epub ahead of print].

24. Pabby A, Schoen RE, Weissfeld JL, et al. Analysis of colorectal cancer occurrence during surveillance colonoscopy in the dietary Polyp Prevention Trial. Gastrointest Endosc 2005;61(3):385–91.

25. Wang YR, Cangemi JR, Loftus EV, et al. Rate of early/missed colorectal cancers after colonoscopy in older patients with and without inflammatory bowel disease in the United States. Am J Gastroenterol 2013;108(3):444–9.

26. Kiesslich R, Fritsch J, Holtmann M, et al. Methylene blue-aided chromoendoscopy for the detection of intraepithelial neoplasia and colon cancer in ulcerative colitis. Gastroenterology 2003;124(4):880–8.

27. Matsumoto T, Nakamura S, Jo Y, et al. Chromoscopy might improve diagnostic accuracy in cancer surveillance for ulcerative colitis. Am J Gastroenterol 2003; 98:1827–33.
28. Rutter MD, Saunders BP, Schofield G, et al. Pancolonic indigo carmine dye spraying for the detection of dysplasia in ulcerative colitis. Gut 2004;53(2): 256–60.
29. Wu L, Li P, Wu J, et al. The diagnostic accuracy of chromoendoscopy for dysplasia in ulcerative colitis: meta-analysis of six randomized controlled trials. Colorectal Dis 2012;14(4):416–20.
30. Subramanian V, Mannath J, Ragunath K, et al. Meta-analysis: the diagnostic yield for detecting dysplasia in patients with colonic inflammatory bowel disease. Aliment Pharmacol Ther 2011;33(3):304–12.
31. Soetikno R, Subramanian V, Kaltenbach T, et al. The detection of nonpolypoid (flat and depressed) colorectal neoplasms in patients with inflammatory bowel disease. Gastroenterology 2013;144(7):1349–52.
32. Sanduleanu S, Rondagh EJ, Masclee AM. Development of expertise in the detection and classification of nonpolypoid colorectal neoplasia: experience-based data at an academic GI unit. Gastrointest Endosc Clin N Am 2010;20:449–60.
33. Rondagh EJ, Bouwens MW, Riedl RG, et al. Endoscopic appearance of proximal colorectal neoplasms and potential implications for colonoscopy in cancer prevention. Gastrointest Endosc 2013;75:1218–25.
34. McGill SK, Kaltenbach T, Friedland S, et al. The learning curve for detection of non-polypoid (flat and depressed) colorectal neoplasms. Gut 2013. [Epub ahead of print].
35. Odze RD, Farraye FA, Hecht JL, et al. Long-term follow-up after polypectomy for adenoma-like dysplastic lesions in ulcerative colitis. Clin Gastroenterol Hepatol 2004;2(7):534–41.
36. Kaltenbach T, Friedland S, Maheshwari A, et al. Short- and long-term outcomes of standardized EMR of nonpolypoid (flat and depressed) colorectal lesions > or = 1cm (with video). Gastrointest Endosc 2007;65(6):857–65.
37. Buchner AM, Guarner-Argente C, Ginsberg GG. Outcomes of EMR of defiant colorectal lesions directed to an endoscopy referral center. Gastrointest Endosc 2012;76(2):255–63.
38. Huang Y, Gong W, Su B, et al. Risk and cause of interval colorectal cancer after colonoscopic polypectomy. Digestion 2012;86:148–54.
39. Gearry RB, Wakeman CJ, Barclay ML, et al. Surveillance for dysplasia in patients with inflammatory bowel disease: a national survey of colonoscopic practice in New Zealand. Dis Colon Rectum 2004;47(3):314–22.
40. van Rijn AF, Fockens P, Siersema PD, et al. Adherence to surveillance guidelines for dysplasia and colorectal carcinoma in ulcerative and Crohn's colitis patients in the Netherlands. World J Gastroenterol 2009;15(2):226–30.
41. Spiegel BM, Ho W, Esrailian E, et al. Controversies in ulcerative colitis: a survey comparing decision making of experts versus community gastroenterologists. Clin Gastroenterol Hepatol 2009;7(2):168–74.
42. Velayos FS, Liu L, Lewis JD, et al. Prevalence of colorectal cancer surveillance for ulcerative colitis in an integrated health care delivery system. Gastroenterology 2010;139(5):1511–8.
43. Robinson RJ, Hart AR, Mayberry JF. Cancer surveillance in ulcerative colitis: a survey of patients' knowledge. Endoscopy 1996;28(9):761–2.
44. Eaden J, Abrams K, Shears J, et al. Randomized controlled trial comparing the efficacy of a video and information leaflet versus information leaflet alone on

patient knowledge about surveillance and cancer risk in ulcerative colitis. Inflamm Bowel Dis 2002;8(6):407–12.

45. Rubio CA. Serrated neoplasia and de novo carcinomas in ulcerative colitis: a histological study in colectomy specimens. J Gastroenterol Hepatol 2007;22(7): 1024–31.

46. Srivastava A, Redson M, Farraye FA, et al. Hyperplastic/serrated polyposis in inflammatory bowel disease: a case series of a previously undescribed entity. Am J Surg Pathol 2008;32(2):296–303.

47. Voorham QJ, Carvalho B, Spiertz AJ, et al. Chromosome 5q loss in colorectal flat adenomas. Clin Cancer Res 2012;18(17):4560–9.

"That Was Me" A Patient's Perspective on Flat Lesion in Inflammatory Bowel Disease

CrossMark

Rachel Zarrow, BA, Alison Zarrow, BA, Hilary Zarrow, JD*

KEYWORDS

- Inflammatory bowel disease • Colonoscopy • Chromoendoscopy • Flat lesion

KEY POINTS

- Flat lesions are often missed on standard colonoscopy.
- Chromoendoscopy is a better detector of flat lesions.

Mr. Z was an active man in his fifties who had worked as an attorney, an investor, and a business advisor. In his free time, he participated in various philanthropies related to health care and housing for the disadvantaged. He exercised, ate a balanced diet, and spent ample time with his wife, 2 daughters, and dogs. On August 31, 2012, he was diagnosed with colon cancer. Four months later, he died. Mr. Z was my father.

Diagnosed with ulcerative colitis at age 19, my dad spent his adult life managing his disease, and following all of his doctors' recommendations. He was closely monitored at expert Inflammatory Bowel Disease centers. He followed the advised gold standard for cancer surveillance, annual colonoscopies.

My dad's ulcerative colitis was considered mild and was limited to a short segment of his left colon. With the help of his doctor and new medications, he rarely had flare ups. Because he considered his disease management a success story, he was happy to give advice to other patients. Over the years, he became the local go-to person for newly diagnosed IBD patients, answering frequent phone calls and questions. He was always upbeat and believed that with proper management his disease would not have to control his life; he had a career and a family, and he still had his colon! His advice to newly diagnosed patients was to find a doctor who was easily accessible and to follow that doctor's recommendations for frequent colonoscopies and vigilance. In order to be a better resource to others, my dad became active in our local Crohn's and Colitis Foundation of America (CCFA) chapter, and he also served on its national board.

Jack and Maxine Zarrow Family Foundation, Tulsa, OK, USA
* Corresponding author. 2120 East 30th Place, Tulsa, OK 74114.
E-mail address: hilzarrow@yahoo.com

Gastrointest Endoscopy Clin N Am 24 (2014) 349–351
http://dx.doi.org/10.1016/j.giec.2014.03.007
1052-5157/14/$ – see front matter © 2014 Elsevier Inc. All rights reserved.

giendo.theclinics.com

Because my dad felt that his disease was cooperating with his treatment, he did not do much independent research on new treatments or colon surveillance protocols followed in other countries. In his mind, there was no need for that; he felt well, and that was all that mattered. His apparent good health was deceiving; unbeknownst to him, his IBD was becoming something malignant.

Until a biopsy from his annual colonoscopy in 2012 showed mild dysplasia, my dad had never heard of a chromoendoscopy, and although he read *The New York Times* daily, he somehow missed the front-page article about chromoendoscopy in March 2008. Had he been having the enhanced surveillance of a chromoendoscopy, as opposed to a colonoscopy, his flat lesion probably would have been detected before it became cancerous, and certainly before it had spread to his lymph nodes and nerves.

According to the current US guidelines and protocol, my father was doing everything right. But the protocol itself is wrong. Traditional white light colonoscopies only detect a fraction of the lesions detectable by chromoendoscopies. The lesion that killed my dad was a flat lesion, one that could have only been detected with a quality chromoendoscopy. In patients with IBD, research shows that chromoendoscopies are better suited to detect flat and depressed lesions. But if patients, especially those suffering from IBD, do not know that this procedure exists, how can they request it of their doctors?

What we have learned from my dad's illness, treatment, and outcome is that patients should enter every doctor's appointment with a critical eye and armed with questions. Before scheduling a colonoscopy and choosing an endoscopist, patients should do their homework. Just as one might research the latest model of a car or washing machine before making an investment, patients should research a potential endoscopist's training and patient outcomes. A few helpful questions[1] might be:

1. In what percentage of patients can you get the endoscope to reach the cecum? (Patients should want endoscopists who reach the cecum in 95% to 98% of patients).
2. What is your adenoma detection rate? (The national benchmark is 25% for men is 25% and 15% for women).
3. How long does the procedure take? (A more thorough test [both in and out] will detect more polyps).
4. Will I get a written report that clearly documents the findings? A good doctor should (1) provide photos of all parts of the colon, (2) comment on bowel preparation, (3) record times (how long the insertion took and the total procedure time), and (4) indicate if he or she examined behind the folds.

Knowing the right questions to ask, my older sister (who also suffers from ulcerative colitis) now has a better handle on her condition. When she first received her diagnosis, our dad assured her that she would be able to manage and live with her disease, just as he had. Because he did not know the questions to ask and did not have annual chromoendoscopies, our dad's illness eventually overtook him. He thought that he was managing his ulcerative colitis when in fact it was silently killing him.

One night in the months leading to his death, our father was awake, looking online at research about his condition. He came across Dr. Roy Soetikno and colleagues'[2] study on chromoendoscopy. Although their findings are very promising for cases such as my sister's, my dad knew that he had come across this research too late. By the time his flat lesion was discovered, it had become invasive cancer. He e-mailed us the link to the article with a short message: "That was me." Armed with the knowledge that a chromoendoscopy could have led to earlier detection of his flat lesion, we now know that the outcome could have been very different. As a family, we are speaking out to doctors and patients alike. Our approach is two-fold. First, we are urging a change in the current US surveillance protocol from colonoscopy with random biopsies to chromoendoscopy with targeted biopsies as the gold standard. Second, we are encouraging patients to research their endoscopist, ask smarter questions, and when appropriate, demand chromoendoscopies over traditional colonoscopies. My dad died, but other IBD patients, my sister included, need not suffer the same fate. The science is there, but it is now up to us to implement it.

REFERENCES

1. Raju GS. Colon cancer screening and prevention. Houston (TX): iTunesU > MD Anderson Cancer Center; 2013. iBook File.
2. Soetikno RM, Kaltenbach T, Rouse RV, et al. Prevalence of nonpolypoid (flat and depressed) colorectal neoplasms in asymptomatic and symptomatic adults. JAMA 2008;299(9):1027–35.

The Potential for Medical Therapy to Reduce the Risk of Colorectal Cancer and Optimize Surveillance in Inflammatory Bowel Disease

Christopher G. Chapman, MD, David T. Rubin, MD*

KEYWORDS

- Medical therapy • Colorectal cancer • Inflammatory bowel disease
- Surveillance endoscopy

KEY POINTS

- Medical therapy, as in the case of 5-aminosalicylic acid, may have mechanistic plausibility for direct antineoplastic properties, but others, such as thiopurines, do not, suggesting that there is a primary chemopreventive benefit derived from the ability to achieve endoscopic and histologic healing.
- Mucosal healing induced by medical therapy may also provide a secondary preventive benefit by allowing improved endoscopic and histologic detection and differentiation between reactive epithelial changes and dysplasia.
- Of the many risk factors for the development of colitis-associated colorectal cancer (CRC), one of the most modifiable for a treating physician is the presence and severity of chronic inflammation.
- Although the mechanism of the declining risk of CRC in IBD is unclear, the likely determinants are a combination of primary prevention resulting from improved medical therapies able to induce mucosal healing, and secondary prevention derived from improved surveillance endoscopy technologies.

INTRODUCTION

Current goals of therapy for inflammatory bowel disease (IBD) are the induction and maintenance of inflammatory symptoms to provide an improved quality of life, to reduce the need for long-term corticosteroids, and to reduce other long-term outcomes such as disability, hospitalization, and colorectal cancer (CRC).[1] Although the success of this latter goal has been difficult to measure, the overall risk of

Inflammatory Bowel Disease Center, University of Chicago Medicine, 5841 South Maryland Avenue, MC 4076, Chicago, IL 60637, USA
* Corresponding author.
E-mail address: drubin@medicine.bsd.uchicago.edu

Gastrointest Endoscopy Clin N Am 24 (2014) 353–365
http://dx.doi.org/10.1016/j.giec.2014.03.008

IBD-associated colorectal cancer (CRC) appears to have declined over the past 30 years.[2] The observed decrease in CRC is thought to be due to a combination of factors, including improvements in the ability to identify and to quantify patients at risk and to detect precancerous lesions, and the direct and indirect reduction in cancer resulting from effective medical and surgical therapies of the underlying inflammation.

Some of the well-defined genetic molecular pathways leading to sporadic or hereditary CRC also appear to be present in colitis-associated CRC. However, IBD-associated adenocarcinoma does not seem to follow the discrete adenoma-to-CRC sequence of events.[3] Rather, a progression, from inflamed mucosa to low-grade dysplasia (LGD) to high-grade dysplasia (HGD) to invasive adenocarcinoma, in IBD remains presumed and unproven. In fact, neoplasia in colitis takes different forms, a fact that has resulted in difficulty classifying, identifying, and developing appropriate prevention strategies for it. Cells from colonic mucosa in patients with chronic colitis have the molecular fingerprints of dysplasia and cancer, including genomic instability (aneuploidy), aberrant DNA methylation, and p53 mutations, even before there is any histologic evidence of dysplasia or cancer.[4] It is thought that such a "field effect" of CRC risk is induced by chronic long-standing mucosal inflammation.

Most recently, the degree of inflammation has been shown to be a significant risk factor for neoplasia in IBD.[5,6] In addition to the presence and degree of severity of active endoscopic/histologic colonic inflammation, additional established IBD-associated dysplasia and CRC risk factors include extent and duration of disease, family history of CRC, concomitant primary sclerosing cholangitis (PSC), young age at diagnosis, and presence of postinflammatory polyps and strictures.[4,6] Of these risks, the only modifiable risk factor may be the degree of active inflammation. Therefore, it has been proposed that effective disease control through abrogation of inflammation may also reduce CRC risk in the individual patient.

Although the culmination of this evidence to date supports the clinician-adopted theory that treating to achieve mucosal healing will reduce the risk of CRC in patients with IBD, it remains uncertain how these recommendations can be practically applied by clinicians trying to develop effective dysplasia and CRC prevention strategies in IBD. This article summarizes the potential for medical therapy to reduce the risk of CRC via primary and secondary prevention, and offers practical ways in which a goal of mucosal improvement or healing may be incorporated into clinical practice (**Box 1**).

DEFINITION OF REMISSION IN IBD: AN EVOLVING TARGET

The end point of escalation of therapy in IBD has traditionally been based on adequate symptom control.[7] Despite patient satisfaction in the achievement of clinical

---

Box 1
Mechanisms by which medical therapy may reduce colorectal cancer in IBD

Primary chemoprevention

  Medical therapy reduces inflammation over time

  Medical therapy has unique chemoprotection mechanisms

Secondary prevention

  Treatment to achieve a healed bowel results in more accurate neoplasia detection by endoscopy

  Reduction in histologic inflammation improves pathologist's diagnosis of neoplasia

remission, in many patients this goal is believed to be insufficient in achieving additional goals of stable remission over time and changing the natural history of the disease. In fact, multiple lines of investigation have demonstrated that a significant proportion of IBD patients in clinical (symptomatic) remission continue to have active mucosal inflammation, both endoscopically and histologically.[8] In addition, a prospective study in patients with active colonic or ileocolonic Crohn's disease treated with steroids found no correlation between the clinical activity index and any of the endoscopic data, and although 92% of patients achieved clinical remission, less than one-third of patients also achieved concomitant endoscopic remission.[9]

Clinically the achievement of a healed mucosa has been associated with a modified course of IBD, including a reduction in rates of clinical relapse, fewer inpatient hospitalizations, and decreased lifetime risk of surgery.[10–12] Evidence that a healed bowel mitigates the development of IBD-associated dysplasia and CRC has been insufficient. With the increased interest in endoscopic mucosal healing in clinical trials, it is hoped that additional evidence will demonstrate a direct link between this end point and subsequent reduction in CRC risk. Clinical trials to date have varied definitions ranging from endoscopic resolution of all mucosal ulcerations to endoscopic scoring indices, with very few studies evaluating histologic healing. Therefore, a remaining challenge is this discrepancy between the clinical trials definition of mucosal healing through endoscopic measures and the available evidence related to risk for neoplasia in colitis, which is histologically measured. More recently, the US Food and Drug Administration has expressed interest in histologic assessment of bowel healing, which undoubtedly will lead to additional study and resource allocation.

Nonetheless, as the bar is raised to achieve deeper levels of mucosal healing, one of the significant challenges is the poor correlation between macroscopic mucosal healing as gauged by endoscopic assessment and endoscopist interpretation, and histologically measured disease control as measured by biopsy sampling and pathologist interpretation. In a study of 152 IBD patients in clinical remission undergoing routine surveillance colonoscopy, Baars and colleagues[8] found that only 67% of patients in clinical remission had histologically active inflammation, and of these patients 50% were endoscopically normal. Similarly, in a study of 82 asymptomatic patients with ulcerative colitis (UC), Rubin and colleagues identified that more than 30% of patients had endoscopic inflammation and 89% had histologic evidence of active inflammation.[13] If it is considered that a strict definition of mucosal healing should include resolution of histologic inflammation in addition to an endoscopic assessment of healing, these studies demonstrate the real-world challenge to this approach and emphasize the importance of further study.

A well-described challenge to the use of mucosal healing as a primary end point of the treatment of IBD is the trade-off between risks and benefits (and costs) in patients who feel well, but require escalation of therapy to achieve deeper levels of disease control. It is unclear whether such additional disease control is possible, and whether patients will be willing to escalate their therapy to achieve such control when they are already in clinical remission. Will such dose or class escalation result in more adverse events than benefits? Will it result, as the available evidence thus far suggests, in most patients "burning" through all of the available therapies and never achieving this level of inflammation control? How will the loss of this level of control and so-called disease drift be monitored? How often, and how invasive will repeated assessments be needed? Obviously there remain many unanswered questions before a disease-wide modification in treatment goals can be applied. Nonetheless, there are ongoing efforts to apply a treat-to-target approach used in other chronic diseases to IBD.[14]

Such paradigm shifts in management will answer these questions and guide future therapies.

TREATMENT TO MUCOSAL HEALING MAY IMPROVE DETECTION OF NEOPLASIA IN IBD

Being able to accurately detect precancerous lesions in patients with colonic IBD is requisite for screening colonoscopy and subsequent interval surveillance examinations. IBD-associated colorectal neoplasia may be a challenge to detect endoscopically because it may be multifocal, broadly infiltrating, and arising from flat mucosa, and therefore endoscopically indistinct from the surrounding tissue. Therefore, to adequately sample representative mucosa and identify dysplasia histologically, historical (and current) guidelines endorsed by multiple societies suggest 4-quadrant random biopsy specimens obtained every 10 cm throughout the colon, aiming to obtain at minimum 32 biopsy samples.[15] However, this approach is limited in that it samples less than 1% of colonic surface area and at the same time is subject to poor patient compliance with surveillance, lack of gastroenterologist knowledge, and compliant practice patterns, in addition to poor pathologist interobserver agreement for dysplasia diagnoses.[16,17]

Furthermore, retrospective studies evaluating the visibility of dysplasia and CRC in patients with IBD have found that most dysplastic lesions are endoscopically visible. In a 14-year, retrospective review of 2204 surveillance colonoscopies, Rutter and colleagues[18] found the neoplastic per-lesion and per-patient sensitivity to be 77.3% and 89.3%, respectively. A total of 22.7% of lesions were macroscopically invisible on colonoscopy. A 10-year, single-institution, retrospective study by Rubin and colleagues[19] in the United States similarly found dysplasia or cancer had per-lesion and per-patient endoscopic visibility of 61.3% and 76.1%, respectively. In this series, 38 of 65 dysplastic lesions (58.5%) and 8 of 10 cancers (80.0%) were visible to the endoscopist as 23 polyps and masses, 1 stricture, and 22 areas of irregular mucosa. In this series 38.7% of lesions were endoscopically invisible, detected only by random biopsy. These retrospective studies did not account for the advent of newer advances in colonoscopic technology, including high-definition or image-enhancement endoscopy techniques such as chromoendoscopy, all of which are believed to further improve visualization and guide future preventive approaches.

In the setting of macroscopically active inflammation, the pathologic diagnosis of dysplasia is often more challenging, primarily because of the difficulty in differentiating inflammation-associated regenerative changes and true dysplasia. In the setting of healing UC, epithelial regeneration occurs with changes that may mimic dysplasia, especially in the eyes of the less experienced pathologist. The epithelial cells become cuboidal with eccentric, large nuclei, mucin depletion, and prominent nucleoli.[20] As a result, pathologists may need to interpret such biopsy specimens as "indefinite for dysplasia" or undiagnosable for dysplasia. Therefore, in addition to the pursuit of mucosal healing as a method of primary prevention of dysplasia and CRC, its achievement may also provide benefit in secondary prevention of CRC, defined as the accurate detection of existing precancerous lesions by gastroenterologists and pathologists. Completing a surveillance colonoscopy in the setting of mucosal healing should improve visualization of neoplastic lesions for the endoscopist, and improve the ability of pathologists to distinguish regenerative change from true dysplasia.

MEDICAL THERAPY AS PRIMARY CHEMOPREVENTION IN IBD-ASSOCIATED NEOPLASIA

The pathophysiology of colitis-associated dysplasia and cancer have implicated the molecular products of chronic inflammation from both innate and adaptive immune cells in the development of a risk-increasing "field effect" of genetic changes in IBD-associated neoplasia.[21] This relationship is supported by the severity of histologic inflammation as an independent risk factor for neoplastic progression.[22,23] In addition to directly reducing inflammation, medical therapy may play a primary chemopreventive role, altering the molecular pathways to dysplasia development (**Box 2**).

5-Aminosalicylates

With demonstrated clinical efficacy and favorable safety profile, 5-aminosalicylic acid (5-ASA) derivatives are the foundational first-line therapy for the induction and maintenance of mild to moderate ulcerative colitis. In addition to the clinical benefit of their anti-inflammatory mechanism, advances in understanding the mechanisms of action reveal multiple molecular chemopreventive properties, including: promotion of cell-cycle arrest to increase the stability of the genome and DNA replication fidelity; inhibition of lipoxygenase and cyclooxygenase-2 (COX-2), thereby regulating angiogenesis via prostaglandin synthesis; scavenging of free radicals and reactive oxygen and nitrogen species to reduce DNA oxidative stress and microsatellite instability; and induction of expression of peroxisome proliferator-activated receptor γ (PPAR-γ), a potent tumor suppressor that interferes with canonical Wnt/β-catenin activity for prevention of CRC.[24–26]

Since 5-ASA was first linked with a reduction in the risk of colitis-associated cancer in 1994,[27] there have been multiple retrospective cohort and case-control observational studies with differing results. In 2005, a systematic review and meta-analysis of 9 observational studies and 1932 patients concluded that there was a protective association between 5-ASA use and cancer (odds ratio [OR] 0.51; 95% confidence interval [CI] 0.37–0.69), and between 5-ASA and cancer and dysplasia (OR 0.51; 95% CI 0.38–0.69).[28] However, since that time, 5 and case-control studies with a larger population cohort have published data that are discordant, demonstrating no protective association.[29–33] The largest of these, using the Manitoba IBD epidemiology database, found no protective benefit in those using 5-ASA therapy for 1 year or longer and 5 years or longer based on a cohort of 8744 IBD patients (OR 1.04, 95% CI 0.67–1.62 and OR 2.01, 95% CI 1.04–3.9, respectively) and a case-control population of 404 CRC patient (OR 1.02, 95% CI 0.60–1.74 and 1.96, 95% CI 0.84–4.55, respectively).[30] Similarly, in a more recent meta-analysis that focused on nonreferral studies to reassess the role of 5-ASA for CRC protection, Nguyen and colleagues[34] found no protective benefit, with a pooled adjusted odds ratio of 0.95 (95% CI 0.66–1.38) and moderate study heterogeneity ($I^2 = 58.2\%$; $P = .07$).

The clinical evidence is hindered by the inherent imperfections of an observational, retrospective investigation, including patient heterogeneity in disease duration and extent, study design and data sources, and monitoring compliance and concomitant medical therapy. There is molecular mechanistic reasoning supporting the use of 5-ASA in colitis-associated cancer prevention, and although the clinical observational studies to date have yielded discrepant results, the 2010 American

---

Box 2
Potential chemoprotective agents in IBD-associated dysplasia and colorectal cancer

5-Aminosalicylic acid

Thiopurine

Anti–tumor necrosis factor antibodies

Gastroenterological Association technical review favored, with moderate certainty, that 5-ASA is chemopreventive against CRC.[35] Although it remains a point of contention, the overall safety of these therapies has resulted in many clinicians continuing their use even when other drugs are used for disease control, even if only because of the possibility of such secondary benefit.

Thiopurines

Systemic immunomodulators including the traditional thiopurines, 6-mercaptopurine (6-MP) and its nitroimidazole derivative, azathioprine (AZA), are purine synthesis inhibitors used in a primary and adjunctive role for the maintenance of remission in patients with both Crohn's disease and UC, in addition to the prevention of immunogenicity against monoclonal antibody therapies, including anti–tumor necrosis factor (TNF)-α and anti-integrin inhibitors. Whereas 5-ASA derivatives have biological mechanisms of action rationalizing their potential role as chemopreventive agents, thiopurines' lack of evidence demonstrating direct antineoplastic mechanisms to suggest any benefit in reducing the risk of dysplasia or CRC may be due to their established anti-inflammatory effects.

Initial studies evaluating the chemopreventive benefits of thiopurines had discrepant results, with most demonstrating no benefit in chemoprevention (but also no increased risk of cancer). In 2010, the available literature was insufficient evidence for the American Gastroenterological Association to make recommendations for or against the use of thiopurines as potential chemopreventive agents.[36] However, recent clinical studies have provided sufficient evidence to reconsider the potential for 6-MP and AZA to reduce the risk of colitis-associated dysplasia and CRC in patients with IBD.

Two large population-based cohorts, similar to prior studies, had different results. In a Dutch cohort of 2578 patients with IBD, van Schaik and colleagues[33] reported that 28 patients (1%) developed HGD or CRC during 16,289 person-years of follow-up. Two of 28 patients (7%) were on thiopurines alone and 1 patient (of 28, 4%) was on a thiopurine plus 5-ASA. Thiopurine use was associated with a significantly decreased risk of developing HGD or CRC with an adjusted hazard ratio (HR) of 0.10 (95% CI 0.01–0.75). However, Pasternak and colleagues[37] found no protective benefit in a Danish cohort of 45,986 IBD patients, of which 11% were on AZA (adjusted relative risk [RR] = 1.00; 95% CI 0.61–1.63).

In 2013, the first prospective study of the epidemiology of colorectal HGD and cancer in IBD in the thiopurine era was published by Beaugerie and colleagues.[38] The results of the CESAME (Cancers Et Surrisque Associé aux Maladies Inflammatoires Intestinales En France) trial, a French nationwide observational cohort of 19,486 patients with IBD designed in the early 2000s to assess the risks of any cancer or HGD in IBD patients, found that 57 (0.3%) patients developed HGD or CRC during the follow-up period (37 CRC, 20 colorectal HGD). In patients with long-standing, extensive colitis, defined as disease duration of at least 10 years and extent of at least 50% of the colon, the multivariate adjusted HR for colorectal HGD and CRC was 0.28 for those who received thiopurines (95% CI 0.1–0.9; $P = .03$).

In the study of inflammation risk by Rubin and colleagues,[5] multivariate analysis identified thiopurine exposure as a significant predictive factor (adjusted OR 0.25; 95% CI 0.08–0.74). This finding, after controlling for degree of inflammation, was one of the strongest lines of evidence to date.

A meta-analysis pooling of 19 studies (9 case-control and 10 cohort studies), while acknowledging high heterogeneity among studies ($I^2 = 68.0\%$, $P<.001$), reported that the use of thiopurine was associated with a statistically significant decreased incidence of CRC or dysplasia (HGD and LGD) with a pooled RR of 0.71 (95% CI 0.54–0.94; P = .017), even after adjustment for duration and extent of the disease.[39] In the thiopurine-treated patients, the RR of HGD and CRC was 0.72 (95% CI 0.50–1.03; P = .070) and 0.70 for CRC (95% CI 0.46–1.09; P = .111).

Despite these recently published reports demonstrating a reduced risk of dysplasia and CRC with thiopurine use, any derived chemopreventive benefit is likely to remain adjunctive to standard clinical indications for use. Given its known risk profile, lack of plausible biological mechanism, success of surveillance colonoscopy, and, possibly, increased anti-inflammatory benefit from anti–TNF-α antibodies, unlike 5-ASA therapies, thiopurines are very unlikely to be recommended as a pure chemopreventive agent in isolation.

Anti–TNF-α Antibodies

Anti-TNF agents are able to induce and maintain mucosal healing in the subset of patients with moderate to severe UC and Crohn's disease, and as a result are likely providing additional chemopreventive benefits by reducing long-standing chronic inflammation. In addition, early investigations into the molecular mechanisms of TNF-α in colitis have suggested a possible direct antineoplastic role from TNF blockade. Using an in vivo dextran sulfate sodium (DSS) and azoxymethane mouse model for chronic colitis–induced cancer, Popivanova and colleagues[40] identified an increase in the levels of TNF-α and infiltrating leukocyte TNF receptor in the colonic mucosa and submucosa before the development of colonic tumors. Treating the mice with a human TNF-α antagonist, etanercept, resulted in decreased tissue injury, and low levels of inflammatory infiltrate and neutrophil-derived and macrophage-derived chemokines. Tumors were reduced in number and size and had poor angiogenesis, presumably from the suppressed COX-2 expression.

The few studies that evaluate the efficacy of anti-TNF agents to reduce the risk of colitis-associated dysplasia and cancer have discordant findings. In a Dutch nationwide, nested case-control study of 173 cases of IBD-associated CRC from 1990 to 2006, the use of anti-TNF (OR 0.09, 95% CI 0.01–0.68; P = .02) was significantly protective for the development of CRC. However, in a nationwide population-based Danish cohort, there was no significant difference in the risk of colitis-associated CRC in IBD-exposed patients when compared with nonexposed patients (adjusted RR 1.06; 95% CI 0.33–3.40).

Ursodeoxycholic Acid

Patients with a concomitant diagnosis of UC and PSC remain at a very high risk for the development of dysplasia and CRC. Ursodeoxycholic acid (UDCA) is a synthetic bile acid that has been proposed to have a molecular mechanism that can reduce the risk of dysplasia and CRC by decreasing the colonic concentration of bile acids, inhibiting Ras gene mutations and COX-2 expression, and having antioxidant activity. In a prospective, randomized, placebo-controlled trial of UDCA therapy in 52 patients with UC and PSC, 10% of patients receiving UDCA developed CRC versus 35% of patients not on UDCA therapy, resulting in a significant RR of 0.26 for developing colorectal dysplasia or cancer (95% CI 0.06–0.92; P = .034).[41] However, this prospective study has been countered by several studies reporting that long-term high-dose (28–30 mg/kg daily) UDCA is not protective in UC or PSC patients, and instead may increase the risk of colorectal neoplasia.[42] Therefore, at present the use of UDCA for chemoprotective reasons alone is not recommended.

A Proposed Approach to the Patient with Ongoing Mucosal Inflammation

With mucosal healing now entrenched as a clinical trial end point and significant evidence demonstrating that mucosal healing modifies the course of the disease, including potentially reducing the risk of cancer via primary and secondary prevention, one question that remains is how is this new paradigm best applied in the clinic? Key issues include how patients in clinical remission should be monitored, and what a clinician should do when active inflammation is encountered on surveillance endoscopy.

Assessment of the mucosa and success at achieving healing requires interval evaluation of the bowel, and current evidence further favors histology. This approach implies the need for repeat endoscopic assessment, which has limitations in cost and patient acceptance. Although endoscopy for dysplasia detection is effective and continually improving with technology, the invasiveness, lack of resources, and, probably, cost-ineffectiveness precludes the performance of endoscopy (and biopsies) every 3 to 6 months from the time of diagnosis. Therefore, surrogate markers of mucosal healing, including blood-based and stool-based biomarkers and noninvasive, nonradiation imaging techniques will remain a focus of continued investigation. For example, the use of neutrophil-derived fecal markers, including calprotectin and lactoferrin, has been positively correlated with endoscopic and histologic activity.[43] The key clinical consideration is that baseline determinations of these noninvasive assessments must be obtained and correlated with endoscopic findings to provide meaning to changes over time. In addition, the timing intervals for monitoring remain unclear. Extrapolating from primary clinical trials evaluating mucosal healing, it is known that in the case of anti–TNF-α agents by week 6 to 8, mucosal healing rates (Mayo endoscopic subscore or equivalent score 0–1) were 42.3% to 62.0% in UC,[41,44–46] and by weeks 10 to 12 were 27% to 31% in Crohn's disease.[47,48] An important point is that in all of the UC trials, the maintenance rates of mucosal healing were all similar to or lower than that at the induction time point, suggesting that surrogate evaluation as frequently as every 8 weeks could indicate a change in mucosal healing.

For now, the most frequent question that arises is related to the performance of routine (guideline-based) surveillance in the asymptomatic patient and the unanticipated inflammation. First, it is important to determine whether the findings are due to an alternative cause such as infection with *Clostridium difficile* or cytomegalovirus. In the setting of true active inflammation, the clinician should reassess the patient's symptoms (or lack thereof) and adherence to the existing regimen of therapy, as often patients will self-discontinue or self-reduce a dose without a discussion with their provider; this is especially true when the patient is feeling well. When patients are truly compliant with therapy and in clinical remission but have endoscopic inflammation, it is reasonable to optimize the existing therapies as an initial step. This approach may include maximizing therapy within the same class of therapies, which can be achieved via therapeutic drug monitoring with thiopurine metabolites or serum monoclonal antibody levels, in addition to determination of antidrug antibodies. After any interval change in therapy, reassessment of the mucosa to determine success is reasonable. The timing of such reassessment is based on the likelihood that a therapeutic adjustment does affect change, which and may occur after 3 to 6 months. Endoscopic or acceptable surrogates may be used to evaluate change. Only after optimization of current therapies has been attempted would it be appropriate to discuss the relative benefits and risks of stepping up to the next class of therapy. Patient acceptance of this approach is critical to implementation (**Box 3**).

A similar approach might be used for patients who desire an alternative or complementary therapy for their IBD. In such unproven therapies, a negotiated trial of the

---

Box 3
Optimization options for the patient who is not healed (without needing to change class of therapy)

Assess Compliance with Current Regimen

5-ASA

    Dose or delivery response

    Increase dose

    Add rectal therapy

Thiopurine

    Assess metabolite profile

    Dose increase

    If shunting, consider allopurinol

Anti-TNF: immunogenicity is a risk

    Dose increase

    Consider levels and antibody assessment

    Switch within class

---

therapy and interval assessment of mucosal healing or other objective benefit can be very helpful for the patient, the clinician, and the so-called therapeutic alliance between them. When such therapeutic trials succeed (or not), an informed discussion about making treatment changes can occur.

FUTURE APPROACHES

Although the incidence of CRC in IBD appears to be decreasing, the mechanism for this decline remains unclear. Significant gaps in the literature remain regarding how clinicians may enhance primary and secondary prevention of colitis-associated dysplasia. There currently is no standard definition of mucosal healing. While clinical trial literature has elected to use any one of the many endoscopic scoring systems, evidence points to persistent histologic inflammation in the setting of endoscopic quiescence. It is theorized that persistent histologic inflammation will increase the risk of CRC, but aggressive efforts to change medical therapy in pursuit of this end point carry both long-term and short-term risks of side effects for an unproven benefit. A unified definition of inflammation control (endoscopic, histologic, radiologic, or other) would allow for better comparison of the efficacy of medical therapy for the induction and maintenance of mucosal healing, in addition to the disease-modifying long-term outcomes, including the risk of colitis-associated CRC.

There is limited to no information about the success of a combination random and targeted surveillance approach to detection of dysplasia, and little has been written about the interval improvement in inflammation control that may also improve detection and prevention. Finally, given the logistical challenges and inherent flaws of retrospective case-control and cohort studies, coupled with the significant number of patients and duration of follow-ups required for prospective CRC prevention studies, it may be best to continue to promote investigation in patient adherence to therapy and compliance to recommended guidelines for surveillance.

In the absence of direct evidence of cancer benefit, the movement of research in IBD toward control of mucosal inflammation as a disease-modifying end point seems sufficient to continue to pursue improved disease control and, secondarily, to anticipate reduced neoplasia as a downstream result.

SUMMARY

Medical therapy, as in the case of 5-ASA, may have mechanistic plausibility for direct antineoplastic properties, but others, such as thiopurines, do not, suggesting that there is a primary chemopreventive benefit derived from the ability to achieve endoscopic and histologic healing. Mucosal healing induced by medical therapy may also provide a secondary preventive benefit by allowing improved endoscopic and histologic detection and differentiation between reactive epithelial changes and dysplasia.

Of the many risk factors for the development of colitis-associated CRC, the only modifiable one for a treating physician is the presence and severity of chronic inflammation. Over the past 20 years, significant progress has been made with the use of agents capable of mucosal healing, and during this time the risk of CRC in IBD patients has declined. Although the mechanism of the declining risk of CRC in IBD remains unclear, the likely determinants are a combination of primary prevention from improved medical therapies able to induce mucosal healing, and secondary prevention from improved surveillance endoscopy technologies.

REFERENCES

1. Kornbluth A, Sachar DB, Practice Parameters Committee of the American College of Gastroenterology. Ulcerative colitis practice guidelines in adults: American College Of Gastroenterology, Practice Parameters Committee. Am J Gastroenterol 2010;105(3):501–23 [quiz: 524].
2. Andersen NN, Jess T. Has the risk of colorectal cancer in inflammatory bowel disease decreased? World J Gastroenterol 2013;19(43):7561–8.
3. Ullman TA, Itzkowitz SH. Intestinal inflammation and cancer. Gastroenterology 2011;140(6):1807–16.
4. Sebastian S, Hernández V, Myrelid P, et al. Colorectal cancer in inflammatory bowel disease: results of the 3rd ECCO pathogenesis scientific workshop (I). J Crohns Colitis 2014;8(1):5–18.
5. Rubin DT, Huo D, Kinnucan JA, et al. Inflammation is an independent risk factor for colonic neoplasia in patients with ulcerative colitis: a case-control study. Clin Gastroenterol Hepatol 2013;11(12):1601–8.e1–4.
6. Rutter MD, Saunders BP, Wilkinson KH, et al. Cancer surveillance in longstanding ulcerative colitis: endoscopic appearances help predict cancer risk. Gut 2004; 53(12):1813–6.
7. Rubin DT. We once were blind and now we see: is it time to treat ulcerative colitis to achieve mucosal healing? Clin Gastroenterol Hepatol 2011;9(6):456–7.
8. Baars JE, Nuij VJ, Oldenburg B, et al. Majority of patients with inflammatory bowel disease in clinical remission have mucosal inflammation. Inflamm Bowel Dis 2012;18(9):1634–40.
9. Modigliani R, Mary JY, Simon JF, et al. Clinical, biological, and endoscopic picture of attacks of Crohn's disease. Evolution on prednisolone. Groupe d'Etude Therapeutique des Affections Inflammatoires Digestives. Gastroenterology 1990;98(4):811–8.
10. Pineton de Chambrun G, Peyrin-Biroulet L, Lémann M, et al. Clinical implications of mucosal healing for the management of IBD. Nat Rev Gastroenterol Hepatol 2010;7(1):15–29.

11. Ardizzone S, Cassinotti A, Duca P, et al. Mucosal healing predicts late outcomes after the first course of corticosteroids for newly diagnosed ulcerative colitis. Clin Gastroenterol Hepatol 2011;9(6):483–9.e3.

12. Froslie KF, Jahnsen J, Moum BA, et al. Mucosal healing in inflammatory bowel disease: results from a Norwegian population-based cohort. Gastroenterology 2007;133(2):412–22.

13. Rubin DT, Koduru P, Surma B, et al. Frequency of Sub-Clinical Disease Activity in Ulcerative Colitis Patients [abstract]. Chicago: DDW 2011.

14. Smolen JS, Aletaha D, Bijlsma JW, et al. Treating rheumatoid arthritis to target: recommendations of an international task force. Ann Rheum Dis 2010;69(4): 631–7.

15. Leighton JA, Shen B, Baron TH, et al. ASGE guideline: endoscopy in the diagnosis and treatment of inflammatory bowel disease. Gastrointest Endosc 2006; 63(4):558–65.

16. Itzkowitz SH, Harpaz N. Diagnosis and management of dysplasia in patients with inflammatory bowel diseases. Gastroenterology 2004;126(6):1634–48.

17. Eaden JA, Ward BA, Mayberry JF. How gastroenterologists screen for colonic cancer in ulcerative colitis: an analysis of performance. Gastrointest Endosc 2000;51(2):123–8.

18. Rutter MD, Saunders BP, Wilkinson KH, et al. Most dysplasia in ulcerative colitis is visible at colonoscopy. Gastrointest Endosc 2004;60(3):334–9.

19. Rubin DT, Rothe JA, Hetzel JT, et al. Are dysplasia and colorectal cancer endoscopically visible in patients with ulcerative colitis? Gastrointest Endosc 2007; 65(7):998–1004.

20. Feldman M, Friedman L, Brandt L. Sleisenger and Fordtran's gastrointestinal and liver disease: pathophysiology, diagnosis, management. 9th edition. Philadelphia: Saunders/Elsevier; 2010.

21. Actis GC, Tarallo S, Rosina F. Cutting edge: chemoprevention of colorectal neoplasia in inflammatory bowel disease. Inflamm Allergy Drug Targets 2013;12(1):1–7.

22. Rutter M, Saunders B, Wilkinson K, et al. Severity of inflammation is a risk factor for colorectal neoplasia in ulcerative colitis. Gastroenterology 2004;126(2): 451–9.

23. Gupta RB, Harpaz N, Itzkowitz S, et al. Histologic inflammation is a risk factor for progression to colorectal neoplasia in ulcerative colitis: a cohort study. Gastroenterology 2007;133(4):1099–105 [quiz: 1340–1].

24. Lyakhovich A, Gasche C. Systematic review: molecular chemoprevention of colorectal malignancy by mesalazine. Aliment Pharmacol Ther 2010;31(2):202–9.

25. Rubin DT, Cruz-Correa MR, Gasche C, et al. Colorectal cancer prevention in inflammatory bowel disease and the role of 5-aminosalicylic acid: a clinical review and update. Inflamm Bowel Dis 2008;14(2):265–74.

26. Subramanian V, Logan RF. Chemoprevention of colorectal cancer in inflammatory bowel disease. Best Pract Res Clin Gastroenterol 2011;25(4–5):593–606.

27. Pinczowski D, Ekbom A, Baron J, et al. Risk factors for colorectal cancer in patients with ulcerative colitis: a case-control study. Gastroenterology 1994; 107(1):117–20.

28. Velayos FS, Terdiman JP, Walsh JM. Effect of 5-aminosalicylate use on colorectal cancer and dysplasia risk: a systematic review and metaanalysis of observational studies. Am J Gastroenterol 2005;100(6):1345–53.

29. Baars JE, Looman CW, Steyerberg EW, et al. The risk of inflammatory bowel disease-related colorectal carcinoma is limited: results from a nationwide nested case-control study. Am J Gastroenterol 2011;106(2):319–28.

30. Bernstein CN, Nugent Z, Blanchard JF. 5-aminosalicylate is not chemoprophy-lactic for colorectal cancer in IBD: a population based study. Am J Gastroenterol 2011;106(4):731–6.

31. Jess T, Loftus EV Jr, Velayos FS, et al. Risk factors for colorectal neoplasia in inflammatory bowel disease: a nested case-control study from Copenhagen county, Denmark and Olmsted county, Minnesota. Am J Gastroenterol 2007; 102(4):829–36.

32. Terdiman JP, Steinbuch M, Blumentals WA, et al. 5-Aminosalicylic acid therapy and the risk of colorectal cancer among patients with inflammatory bowel disease. Inflamm Bowel Dis 2007;13(4):367–71.

33. van Schaik FD, van Oijen MG, Smeets HM, et al. Thiopurines prevent advanced colorectal neoplasia in patients with inflammatory bowel disease. Gut 2012;61(2): 235–40.

34. Nguyen GC, Gulamhusein A, Bernstein CN, et al. 5-aminosalicylic acid is not protective against colorectal cancer in inflammatory bowel disease: a meta-analysis of non-referral populations. Am J Gastroenterol 2012;107:1298–304.

35. Farraye FA, Odze RD, Eaden J, et al. AGA technical review on the diagnosis and management of colorectal neoplasia in inflammatory bowel disease. Gastroenterology 2010;138(2):746–74, 774.e1–4. [quiz: e12–3].

36. Farraye FA, Odze RD, Eaden J, et al. AGA medical position statement on the diagnosis and management of colorectal neoplasia in inflammatory bowel disease. Gastroenterology 2010;138(2):738–45.

37. Pasternak B, Svanström H, Schmiegelow K, et al. Use of azathioprine and the risk of cancer in inflammatory bowel disease. Am J Epidemiol 2013;177(11): 1296–305.

38. Beaugerie L, Svrcek M, Seksik P, et al. Risk of colorectal high-grade dysplasia and cancer in a prospective observational cohort of patients with inflammatory bowel disease. Gastroenterology 2013;145(1):166–75.e8.

39. Gong J, Zhu L, Guo Z, et al. Use of thiopurines and risk of colorectal neoplasia in patients with inflammatory bowel diseases: a meta-analysis. PLoS One 2013; 8(11):e81487.

40. Popivanova BK, Kitamura K, Wu Y, et al. Blocking TNF-alpha in mice reduces colorectal carcinogenesis associated with chronic colitis. J Clin Invest 2008; 118(2):560–70.

41. Pardi DS, Loftus EV Jr, Kremers WK, et al. Ursodeoxycholic acid as a chemopreventive agent in patients with ulcerative colitis and primary sclerosing cholangitis. Gastroenterology 2003;124(4):889–93.

42. Eaton JE, Silveira MG, Pardi DS, et al. High-dose ursodeoxycholic acid is associated with the development of colorectal neoplasia in patients with ulcerative colitis and primary sclerosing cholangitis. Am J Gastroenterol 2011;106(9):1638–45.

43. Vieira A, Fang CB, Rolim EG, et al. Inflammatory bowel disease activity assessed by fecal calprotectin and lactoferrin: correlation with laboratory parameters, clinical, endoscopic and histological indexes. BMC Res Notes 2009;2:221.

44. Rutgeerts P, Sandborn WJ, Feagan BG, et al. Infliximab for induction and maintenance therapy for ulcerative colitis. N Engl J Med 2005;353(23):2462–76.

45. Sandborn WJ, Feagan BG, Marano C, et al. Subcutaneous golimumab induces clinical response and remission in patients with moderate-to-severe ulcerative colitis. Gastroenterology 2014;146(1):85–95 [quiz: e14–5].

46. Sandborn WJ, van Assche G, Reinisch W, et al. Adalimumab induces and maintains clinical remission in patients with moderate-to-severe ulcerative colitis. Gastroenterology 2012;142(2):257–65.e1–3.

47. Rutgeerts P, Diamond RH, Bala M, et al. Scheduled maintenance treatment with infliximab is superior to episodic treatment for the healing of mucosal ulceration associated with Crohn's disease. Gastrointest Endosc 2006;63(3): 433–42 [quiz: 464].
48. Rutgeerts P, van Assche G, Sandborn WJ, et al. Adalimumab induces and maintains mucosal healing in patients with Crohn's disease: data from the EXTEND trial. Gastroenterology 2012;142(5):1102–11.e2.

Mucosal Healing As a Target of Therapy for Colonic Inflammatory Bowel Disease and Methods to Score Disease Activity

 CrossMark

Alissa Walsh, FRACP[a], Rebecca Palmer, MRCP[b],
Simon Travis, DPhil, FRCP[b],*

KEYWORDS

- Mucosal healing • Ulcerative colitis • Crohn's disease • Inflammatory bowel disease

KEY POINTS

- Mucosal healing is an important end point in clinical trials.
- Mucosal healing predicts the following:
  - Less corticosteroid use
  - Lower hospitalization rates
  - Increased sustained clinical remission
  - Lower colectomy and bowel resection rates
- Mucosal healing decreases the risk of colorectal cancer in ulcerative colitis (UC).
- Mucosal healing should be recognized by clinicians and health care providers as a goal for inflammatory bowel disease (IBD) therapy.

INTRODUCTION

UC and Crohn's disease are characterized by the presence of gut inflammation accompanied by areas of ulceration (**Fig. 1**). Mucosal healing is becoming increasingly important in the clinical management of UC and Crohn's disease, as well as being used as an end point in clinical trials. Achieving mucosal healing has unequivocally been associated with better outcomes, and for these reasons, it has become an important treatment goal. There are, however, multiple methods to score endoscopic disease activity in both UC and Crohn's disease. This article therefore focuses on

[a] Gastroenterology Department, St Vincent's Hospital, 390 Victoria Street, Darlinghurst, Sydney NSW 2010, Australia; [b] Translational Gastroenterology Unit, John Radcliffe Hospital, Oxford OX3 9DU, UK
* Corresponding author.
E-mail address: Simon.Travis@ndm.ox.ac.uk

Gastrointest Endoscopy Clin N Am 24 (2014) 367–378
http://dx.doi.org/10.1016/j.giec.2014.03.005
1052-5157/14/$ – see front matter © 2014 Elsevier Inc. All rights reserved.

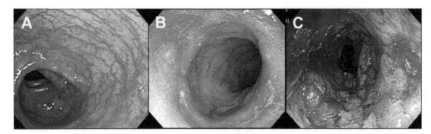

Fig. 1. Assessment of mucosal healing using the Ulcerative Colitis Endoscopic Index of Severity (UCEIS) with descriptors of vascular pattern (V), bleeding (B), and erosions/ulcers (E). (*A*) UCEIS 0 (V0 B0 E0), (*B*) UCEIS 5 (V2 B1 E0), and (*C*) UCEIS 8 (V2 B3 E3).

those used most frequently or that have been validated: the Mayo endoscopic score and the Ulcerative Colitis Endoscopic Index of Severity (UCEIS) for UC and the Crohn's Disease Endoscopic Index of Severity (CDEIS), the Simple Endoscopic Score for Crohn's Disease (SES-CD), and the Rutgeerts Postoperative Endoscopic Index for Crohn's disease. Because indices are complex and potentially confusing, the article follows a standard approach describing the indices in this order.

DEFINITION OF MUCOSAL HEALING

Mucosal healing in the context of IBD refers to the endoscopic assessment of disease activity. Simply stated, mucosal healing should imply the absence of ulceration and erosions. Nevertheless, there is currently no validated definition of mucosal healing in IBD.[1–3]

Ulcerative Colitis

In patients with UC, mucosal healing may represent the ultimate therapeutic goal, because the disease is limited to the mucosa. The pattern of inflammation in UC is associated with several mucosal changes, initially vascular congestion, erythema, and granularity. As inflammation becomes more severe, friability (bleeding to light touch), spontaneous bleeding, and erosions and ulcers develop. An International Organization of Inflammatory Bowel Disease (IOIBD) task force defined mucosal healing in UC as the absence of friability, blood, erosions, and ulcers in all visualized segments of the colonic mucosa.[2] However, some studies allow erythema and friability in the definition of mucosal healing.[4] Many different endoscopic indices for UC have been used in clinical trials, although none have been fully validated in prospective studies; this creates problems when comparing trials.[5]

Crohn's Disease

In contrast to UC, mucosal healing in Crohn's disease might reasonably be considered a minimum (rather than the ultimate) therapeutic goal, because the disease is transmural. Even this therapeutic goal, however, is not routine clinical practice in most centers. The pattern of inflammation in Crohn's disease is characterized by several mucosal features that include patchy erythema, nodularity, aphthoid, and then deeper, serpiginous ulceration, strictures, and, in severe cases, penetrating ulcers. The complete resolution of all visible ulcers is a simple definition of mucosal healing for clinical practice, and this is what has been suggested by IOIBD task force.[6] Nevertheless, this binomial definition (presence or absence of ulcers) is currently unvalidated, is difficult to achieve, and is rather crude for use in therapeutic trials because it does not allow quantification of improvement of mucosal inflammation.[7] The largest trials that have used mucosal healing as a primary or major secondary end point have used the definition of absence of ulcers rather than the prespecified cut-off values on the CDEIS or SES-CD. Studies have yet to determine the minimum degree of endoscopic improvement associated with improved clinical outcomes.

BENEFITS OF MUCOSAL HEALING

Mucosal healing in IBD has been associated with the following:

- Decreased need for corticosteroids[8]
- Decreased hospitalization rates[9–11]
- Sustained clinical remission[11,12]
- Decreased colectomy and bowel resection[5,8,9,11,12]
- Decreased risk of colorectal cancer[13]

Multivariate analysis of data from a case-controlled study of patients with long-standing, extensive UC showed that those with endoscopically normal mucosa at surveillance colonoscopy had the same 5-year cancer risk as the general population.[13] The presence of persisting histologic inflammation was, however, a determinant of risk for colorectal cancer.[14] In the same surveillance population, evidence of postinflammatory polyps or strictures was associated with a significantly increased colorectal cancer risk. For Crohn's disease, there has been no demonstrable reduction in colorectal cancer in those with mucosal healing.

Before monoclonal antibodies against tumor necrosis factor (anti-TNF) were introduced for Crohn's disease, a symptom-oriented management approach was common. This approach was largely used because of the failure to demonstrate a correlation between endoscopic remission (mucosal healing) and decrease in relapse rates in patients treated with steroids compared with clinical remission (symptom control). Steroids, however, do not heal the ileal or colonic mucosa. In contrast, both azathioprine and anti-TNF therapy have now been shown to achieve and then maintain mucosal healing, thereby influencing the course of Crohn's disease.[8,10]

For these reasons, mucosal healing has emerged since 2012 as an important therapeutic goal for both UC and Crohn's disease. Moreover, because trials in IBD have traditionally had a high placebo response rate, there is a move to include mucosal healing as an end point in trials to drive down placebo rates.[15,16] For most patients, mucosal healing is only maintained with continued therapy. Current treatments do not cure the disease, and therefore, cessation of therapy almost invariably leads to disease recurrence.[17] If mucosal healing influences the subsequent course of disease, logic suggests that its presence should be confirmed or therapy augmented if it has not been achieved. For these reasons, endoscopic assessment is increasingly used in clinical practice to guide decision making in the management of IBD, but augmenting treatment in the absence of symptoms just because endoscopic lesions are present remains a challenge to many clinicians. On the other hand, most are persuaded that mucosal healing is an appropriate therapeutic goal when starting, stepping up, switching, or stopping expensive biologic therapy.

LIMITATIONS OF MUCOSAL HEALING

Although colonoscopy is considered to be a low-risk invasive procedure, it still carries a risk of perforation, bleeding, or sedation. Furthermore, colonoscopy is an investment of time and resources both for the patient and the community.

Even when using validated indices such as the UCEIS and CDEIS, further research is needed to determine what degree of improvement, measured by endoscopy, is clinically meaningful. In addition, although disease may seem inactive at endoscopy, microscopic disease activity may persist. Persistent histologic activity is associated with a shorter time to relapse in UC,[18,19] so endoscopic mucosal healing alone may be an insufficient therapeutic goal.[20] Surrogate, noninvasive markers of mucosal healing are therefore needed, but biomarkers such as fecal calprotectin have yet to demonstrate sufficient specificity for mucosal healing to replace endoscopic assessment.[17]

METHODS TO SCORE DISEASE ACTIVITY
Ulcerative Colitis

Truelove and Witts[21] were the first to comment on mucosal appearance as a measure of disease activity, using rigid sigmoidoscopy in the first placebo-controlled trial of cortisone for UC in 1955. Since 1956, it has been recognized that endoscopic and histologic microscopic changes can persist despite symptom resolution.[22] Endoscopic indices evolved from the Baron score,[23] initially developed for rigid proctoscopy in ambulatory patients with mild to moderate disease, which rated vascular pattern, mucosal bleeding, and friability. Subsequent endoscopic indices of increasing complexity incorporated the presence of ulcers, mucopus, granularity, and appearance of light scattering, in addition to bleeding and friability. Such modifications were intended to improve the capture of disease activity, but they invariably increased the subjectivity of the scoring system. **Table 1** summarizes commonly used endoscopic indices for UC, none of which have been validated with the exception of the UCEIS.[31] Nonetheless, there is no agreed threshold for defining either mucosal healing or endoscopic remission, which makes it almost impossible to compare mucosal healing rates between studies.[33]

Space does not allow a review of all indices, so this article focuses on the Mayo Clinic endoscopy subscore, because this is commonly used in clinical trials, and the UCEIS, which has been validated.

The Mayo Clinic endoscopy subscore has 4 components, with a maximum total score of 3 (**Table 2**).[26] There is overlap in the features of the different levels of this endoscopic index, which causes high interobserver variation. The most troublesome component of this index is friability, as this is subjective and leads to inconsistent results.[34] This inconsistency has lead to an adaptation of the index to remove friability from level 1.[35]

The value of this index lies with its widespread use in clinical trials. In trials of infliximab and adalimumab, mucosal healing was defined as a Mayo subscore of 0 or 1 or a decrease from the baseline subscores of 2 or 3. In Active Ulcerative Colitis Trials, patients with a posttreatment Mayo score of grade 1 were no more likely to undergo a colectomy than those with a score of 0.[36]

The UCEIS (**Table 3**) was developed because of wide interobserver variation in endoscopic assessment of disease activity.[31] There was only 76% agreement for severe and 27% agreement for normal endoscopic mucosal appearances between 10 experienced investigators and a central reader. Thirty different investigators then rated 25/60 different videos for 10 descriptors and assessed overall severity on a 0 to 100 visual analog scale. Kappa statistics tested interobserver and intraobserver variability for each descriptor. Different models to predict the overall assessment of severity as judged by a visual analog scale were developed using general linear mixed regression. The final model incorporated just 3 descriptors, each with precise definitions. A third validation phase used another 25 different investigators from North America and Europe, who assessed in a randomly selected subset of 28/60 videos, including

Table 1
Endoscopic disease activity indices[a] for ulcerative colitis

Index[a]	Validated	Variables	Strengths	Weaknesses
Truelove and Witts Endoscopy Index[21]	No	Granularity, hyperemia	Precedence (first reported index), but no other merit	No description of endoscopic lesions, so interobserver variability is high
Baron Index[23]	No	Bleeding, vascular pattern, friability	Easy to use	Ulcerations not included in score, no definition of mucosal healing
Powell-Tuck Index[24]	No	Bleeding	Easy to use	Ulceration not included, no definition of mucosal healing
Sutherland Index[25]	No	Friability, bleeding, exudation	Easy to use; overlap in descriptive terms used for different levels of activity	Subjective, no definition of mucosal healing
Mayo Clinic Index: endoscopic subscore[26]	No	Vascular pattern, erythema, friability, erosions and ulcerations, bleeding	Easy to use, commonly used in clinical trials; overlap in descriptive terms used for different levels of activity	No validated definition of mucosal healing. The term minimal or slight friability is subjective and leads to inconsistent results
Rachmilewitz Index[27]	No	Granulation, mucosal damage, vascular pattern, vulnerability of mucosa (bleeding)	None reported	Complex and subjective descriptive terms
Modified Baron Index[28]	No	Vascular pattern, granularity, friability, bleeding, ulceration	Easy to use	No validated definition of mucosal healing
Endoscopic Activity Index[29]	No	Size of ulcers (4 levels), depth of ulcers (4 levels), redness (3 levels), Bleeding (4 levels), mucosal edema (4 levels), mucosal exudate (3 levels)	Closely correlated with clinical activity. Comparable to other indices. Useful in severe disease	
Matts Index[30]	No	Granularity, bleeding, edema, ulceration	Easy to use	
Ulcerative Colitis Endoscopic Index or Severity[31]	Preliminary[32]	Vascular pattern (3 levels), bleeding (4 levels), ulceration (4 levels)	Easy to use. Independent of clinical symptoms, accounts for 88% of variation between observers	Sensitivity to change, and mucosal healing remain undefined

[a] The word index is best used for an instrument designed to assess activity and score for the level of activity assigned by the index.[31]

Table 2
Mayo endoscopic score

Score	Disease Activity	Endoscopic Features (Descriptors)
0	Normal or inactive	None
1	Mild	Erythema, decreased vascular pattern, mild friability[a]
2	Moderate	Marked erythema, absent vascular pattern, friability, erosions
3	Severe	Spontaneous bleeding, ulceration

[a] Endoscopic assessment in the mesalamine MMX trials removed friability from level 1 (see text).
Adapted from Schroeder KW, Tremaine WJ, Ilstrup DM. Coated oral 5-aminosalicylic acid therapy for mildly to moderately active ulcerative colitis. A randomized study. N Engl J Med 1987;317:1625–9; with permission.

2 duplicated videos to assess test-retest reliability. Intraobserver kappa values were 0.82, 0.72, and 0.78 for vascular pattern, bleeding, and erosion and ulcer descriptors, and interobserver kappa values were 0.83, 0.56, and 0.77, respectively. The correlation coefficient (r^2) between UCEIS and overall severity evaluation was 0.94 ($P<.0001$), meaning that it accounted for 88% (0.94^2) of the variation between observers in the overall assessment of endoscopic activity.[32]

The term friability invariably needs explanation. The UCEIS dispensed with the term mucosal friability, because the model including friability as a descriptor did not

Table 3
The Ulcerative Colitis Endoscopic Index of Severity

Descriptor (Score Most Severe Lesions)	Likert Scale Anchor Points	Definition
Vascular pattern	Normal (0)	Normal vascular pattern with arborization of capillaries clearly defined, or with blurring or patchy loss of capillary margins
	Patchy obliteration (1)	Patchy obliteration of vascular pattern
	Obliterated (2)	Complete obliteration of vascular pattern
Bleeding	None (0)	No visible blood
	Mucosal (1)	Some spots or streaks of coagulated blood on the surface of the mucosa ahead of the scope, which can be washed away
	Luminal mild (2)	Some free liquid blood in the lumen
	Luminal moderate or severe (3)	Frank blood in the lumen ahead of endoscope or visible oozing from mucosa after washing intraluminal blood, or visible oozing from a hemorrhagic mucosa
Erosions and ulcers	None (0)	Normal mucosa, no visible erosions or ulcers
	Erosions (1)	Tiny ($\leq$5 mm) defects in the mucosa, of a white or yellow color with a flat edge
	Superficial ulcer (2)	Larger (>5 mm) defects in the mucosa, which are discrete fibrin-covered ulcers when compared with erosions, but remain superficial
	Deep ulcer (3)	Deeper excavated defects in the mucosa, with a slightly raised edge

Copyright Warner Chilcott Pharmaceuticals, although the index is freely available for use by investigators.
Adapted from Neurath MF, Travis SP. Mucosal healing in inflammatory bowel diseases: a systematic review. Gut 2012;61:1619–35.

perform significantly better than one including bleeding. In practical terms, the most severely affected part of the mucosa is scored. There are, however, still limitations; thresholds for remission and mild, moderate, and severe disease have yet to be set. The extent to which full colonoscopy may influence the score compared with the flexible sigmoidoscopy on which it was based, has only started to be evaluated.[37] Knowledge of symptoms does not materially influence the score, and a comparison with the Mayo Clinic endoscopy subscore shows that the UCEIS is less subject to variation by a central reader.[38] Nevertheless, the UCEIS is simple enough to use in clinical practice and should achieve its goal of reducing variation in endoscopic assessment of activity between observers. Clinicians are beginning to use the UCEIS in clinical practice, and a preliminary study in patients admitted with acute severe colitis shows that a score of 7 or 8 (out of 8) on admission predicted an inadequate response to intravenous steroids and the need for rescue therapy with cyclosporine or infliximab.[39] The UCEIS is now being used in clinical trials of UC that are in progress.

Crohn's Disease

There are validated endoscopic indices for the assessment of Crohn's disease activity (**Table 4**). The CDEIS is the standard, whereas the SES-CD is a simplified version. The Rutgeerts Postoperative Endoscopic Index is used for estimating the risk of recurrence after ileocolic resection for Crohn's disease.

The CDEIS[40] is a prospectively developed instrument constructed to detect changes in disease activity and examines 4 endoscopic variables (deep ulceration, superficial ulceration, length of ulcerated mucosa, and length of diseased mucosa) in each of the following locations: rectum, sigmoid and left colon, transverse colon, and right colon and ileum (**Table 5**). The total score is then divided by the number

Table 4
Endoscopic indices for Crohn's disease

Index	Validated	Variables	Strengths	Weaknesses
Crohn's Disease Endoscopic Index of Severity (CDEIS)[40]	Yes	Superficial and deep ulceration, ulcerated and nonulcerated stenosis, surface area of ulcerated and disease segments	Standard, reproducible, gold standard	Complex, need experience/ training, difficult for beginners and daily routine, no validated definition of mucosal healing
Simple Endoscopic Score for Crohn's Disease (SES-CD)[41]	Yes	Ulcer size, ulcerated surface, affected surface, presence of stenosis	Simplified index; performance correlates with CDEIS	Validated against CDEIS in only one study, less frequently used than CDEIS, no validated definition of mucosal healing
Rutgeerts Postoperative Endoscopic Index[42]	No	Aphthous ulcerations, inflammation, ulcers, nodules, narrowing	Standard for evaluating postoperative recurrence, validated levels for predicting relapse	Only for use after ileocolic resection

Table 5
Example of the CDEIS scoring form

	Rectum	Sigmoid & Left Colon	Transverse Colon	Right Colon	Ileum	Total	
Deep ulcerations (12 present, 0 absent)	0	12	0	12	N/A	24	Total 1
Superficial ulceration (6 present, 0 absent)	6	6	6	6	N/A	24	Total 2
Surface involved by the disease (per 10 cm)[a]	5.6	4.9	3.4	5.6	N/A	19.5	Total 3
Ulcerated surface (per 10 cm)[a]	0.7	0.5	0.9	0.4	N/A	22	Total 4
Total 1 + Total 2 + Total 3 + Total 4						89.5	Total A
Number (n) of segments totally or partially examined (1–5)						4	n
Total A divided by n						22.4	Total B
Quote 3 if ulcerated stenosis anywhere, 0 if not						3	C
Quote 3 if nonulcerated stenosis anywhere, 0 if not						0	D
Total B + C + D						25.4	CDEIS

[a] Analog scales to be converted to numeric values.
Adapted from Mary JY, Modigliani R. Development and validation of an endoscopic index of the severity for Crohn's disease: a prospective multicentre study. Groupe d'Etudes Thérapeutiques des Affections Inflammatoires du Tube Digestif (GETAID). Gut 1989;30:983–9; with permission.

of locations explored (1–5). An additional 3 points is given if an ulcerated stenosis is present, and a further 3 points if a nonulcerated stenosis is present. CDEIS scores range from 0 to 44.

- Deep ulcerations: score 0 if absent or 12 if present
- Superficial ulcerations: score 0 if absent or 6 if present
- Length of ulcerated mucosa (0–10 cm): score 0 to 10 according to length in centimeters
- Length of diseased mucosa (0–10 cm): score 0 to 10 according to length in centimeters

Although CDEIS is the standard index and is reproducible, it is also complex. It requires training and experience, especially for estimating ulcerated or diseased mucosal surfaces and distinguishing between superficial and deep ulceration. It is cumbersome to use in clinical practice. The CDEIS has appropriate sensitivity to measure changes in the mucosal appearance. Endoscopic remission (minor or no lesions) is defined as a CDEIS score less than or equal to 6 or less than or equal to 7, and complete endoscopic remission (mucosal healing, ie, no lesions at all or scarred lesions only) is defined as a CDEIS score less than or equal to 3 or less than or equal to 4. An endoscopic response is a decrease from baseline CDEIS score of at least 4 or 5 points. The CDEIS has been used in trials of corticosteroids, thiopurines, and TNF antagonists.

In the MUSIC (Endoscopic Mucosal Improvement in Patients With Active Crohn's Disease Treated With Certolizumab Pegol) study of certolizumab pegol in Crohn's disease, maintenance of improvement between weeks 10 and 54, based on individual patient data, was found in 70% of those who responded (decline in CDEIS >5) and those with complete remission (CDEIS<3), and in more than 40% of those with remission (CDEIS<6).[43]

The SES-CD (**Table 6**) correlates well with the CDEIS, with a correlation coefficient r = 0.920 and excellent interobserver reliability (k coefficients 0.791–1.000). This score

Table 6
Simple Endoscopic Score for Crohn's Disease

Variable	0	1	2	3
Size of ulcers (cm)	None	Aphthous ulcers (diameter 0.1–0.5 cm)	Large ulcers (diameter 0.5–2 cm)	Very large ulcers (diameter >2 cm)
Ulcerated surface (%)	None	<10	10–30	>30
Affected surface (%)	Unaffected segment	<50	50–75	>75
Presence of narrowings	None	Single, can be passed	Multiple, can be passed	Cannot be passed

Total SES-CD: sum of the values of the 4 variables for the 5 bowel segments. Values are given to each variable and for every examined bowel segment.

Adapted from Daperno M, D'Haens G, Van Assche G, et al. Development and validation of a new, simplified endoscopic activity score for Crohn's disease: the SES-CD. Gastrointest Endosc 2004;60:505–12; with permission.

was developed to meet the need for a reliable, easy-to-use endoscopic scoring instrument for Crohn's disease, one that by contrast would be less complex than the CDEIS. Selected endoscopic parameters (ulcer size, ulcerated and affected surfaces, stenosis) were scored from 0 to 3, whereby SES-CD = 0 equates to absence of ulcers.[41] No cutoff values have been determined for the SES-CD, and there is no definition of mucosal healing.

The Rutgeerts Postoperative Endoscopic Index (**Table 7**) determines the severity of endoscopic disease recurrence at the anastomosis and in the neoterminal ileum after ileocolic resection.[42,44] The severity of endoscopic recurrence predicts clinical recurrence, so it has gained popularity.[42] In the year after ileocolic resection, patients with a Rutgeerts score of 0 or 1 have a low risk of clinical recurrence (20% at 3 years follow-up) compared with those patients who have a score of grade 3 or 4 (92% at 3 years follow-up). Level 2 is associated with an intermediate risk of clinical recurrence, but the definition of grade 2 is more subjective and is exposed to variability.

This index has also been incorporated into a randomized clinical trial. In the Post Operative Crohn's Endoscopic Recurrence study, it was shown that treating according to the risk of recurrence with a 6-month postoperative colonoscopy and treatment

Table 7
Rutgeerts Postoperative Endoscopic Index

	Distal Ileum
Grade 0	Nil
Grade 1	≤5 Aphthous ulcers
Grade 2	>5 Aphthous ulcers with normal intervening mucosa, or skip areas of larger lesions or lesions confined to the ileocolic anastomosis (ie, <1 cm in length)
Grade 3	Diffuse aphthous ulceration with diffusely inflamed mucosa
Grade 4	Diffuse inflammation with large ulcers, nodules, and/or narrowing

An endoscopic scoring system for postoperative disease recurrence in Crohn's disease. The original paper uses the term grade rather than level, and as with other tables, the descriptions are precisely those used in the original paper.

Adapted from Rutgeerts P, Geboes K, Vantrappen G, et al. Predictability of the postoperative course of Crohn's disease. Gastroenterology 1990;99:956–63; with permission.

step up for those who had a Rutgeerts score $\geq$i2, is significantly superior to drug therapy alone in preventing postoperative recurrence.[45]

SUMMARY

The colonoscopic assessment of mucosal healing has proved increasingly important in the management of both UC and Crohn's disease. All clinicians should strive for this goal. There is evidence for a decrease in corticosteroid use, decreased hospitalization, an increase in sustained remission, and a decrease in the need for surgery. Further advancements with surrogate noninvasive markers for mucosal healing may help to overcome existing limitations and need for colonoscopy. Multiple endoscopic indices exist for UC; however, the only validated index is the UCEIS, and its use in both clinical practice and clinical trials is encouraged. The CDEIS and the SES-CD are both validated for Crohn's disease. The Rutgeerts Postoperative Endoscopic Index is useful for the prediction of postoperative recurrence in those patients who have had an ileocolic resection.

REFERENCES

1. Sandborn WJ, Feagan BG, Hanauer SB, et al. A review of activity indices and efficacy end points for clinical trials of medical therapy in adults with Crohn's disease. Gastroenterology 2002;122(2):512–30.
2. D'Haens G, Sandborn WJ, Feagan BG, et al. A review of activity indices and efficacy end points for clinical trials of medical therapy in adults with ulcerative colitis. Gastroenterology 2007;132(2):763–86.
3. Neurath MF, Travis SP. Mucosal healing in inflammatory bowel diseases: a systematic review. Gut 2012;61(11):1619–35.
4. Dave M, Loftus EV. Mucosal healing in inflammatory bowel disease - a true paradigm of success? Gastroenterol Hepatol 2012;8(1):29–38.
5. Walsh AJ, Ghosh A, Brain AO, et al. Comparing disease activity indices in ulcerative colitis. J Crohns Colitis 2014;8:318–25.
6. D'Haens GR, Fedorak R, Lémann M, et al. End points for clinical trials evaluating disease modification and structural damage in adults with Crohn's disease. Inflamm Bowel Dis 2009;15(10):1599–604.
7. De Cruz P, Kamm MA, Prideaux L, et al. Mucosal healing in Crohn's disease: a systematic review. Inflamm Bowel Dis 2013;19(2):429–44.
8. Frøslie KF, Jahnsen J, Moum BA, et al. Mucosal healing in inflammatory bowel disease: results from a Norwegian population-based cohort. Gastroenterology 2007;133(2):412–22.
9. Ardizzone S, Maconi G, Russo A, et al. Randomised controlled trial of azathioprine and 5-aminosalicylic acid for treatment of steroid dependent ulcerative colitis. Gut 2006;55(1):47–53.
10. Rutgeerts P, Diamond RH, Bala M, et al. Scheduled maintenance treatment with infliximab is superior to episodic treatment for the healing of mucosal ulceration associated with Crohn's disease. Gastrointest Endosc 2006;63(3):433–42.
11. Schnitzler F, Fidder H, Ferrante M, et al. Mucosal healing predicts long-term outcome of maintenance therapy with infliximab in Crohn's disease. Inflamm Bowel Dis 2009;15(9):1295–301.
12. Colombel JF, Rutgeerts P, Reinisch W, et al. Early mucosal healing with infliximab is associated with improved long-term clinical outcomes in ulcerative colitis. Gastroenterology 2011;141(4):1194–201.

13. Rutter MD, Saunders BP, Wilkinson KH, et al. Cancer surveillance in longstanding ulcerative colitis: endoscopic appearances help predict cancer risk. Gut 2004; 53(12):1813–6.
14. Rutter M, Saunders B, Wilkinson K, et al. Severity of inflammation is a risk factor for colorectal neoplasia in ulcerative colitis. Gastroenterology 2004;126(2): 451–9.
15. Rutgeerts P, Van Assche G, Sandborn WJ, et al. Adalimumab induces and maintains mucosal healing in patients with Crohn's disease: data from the EXTEND trial. Gastroenterology 2012;142(5):1102–11.e2.
16. De Cruz P, Bernardi MP, Kamm MA, et al. Postoperative recurrence of Crohn's disease: impact of endoscopic monitoring and treatment step-up. Colorectal Dis 2013;15(2):187–97.
17. Schoepfer AM, Vavricka S, Zahnd-straumann N, et al. Monitoring inflammatory bowel disease activity: clinical activity is judged to be more relevant than endoscopic severity or biomarkers. J Crohns Colitis 2012;6(4):412–8.
18. Riley SA, Mani V, Goodman MJ, et al. Microscopic activity in ulcerative colitis: what does it mean? Gut 1991;32(2):174–8.
19. Burger DC, Thomas SJ, Walsh AJ, et al. Depth of remission may not predict outcome of UC over 2 years. Gut 2011;60(Suppl 1):A133.
20. Peyrin-Biroulet L, Bressenot A, Kampman W. Histologic remission: the ultimate therapeutic goal in ulcerative colitis? Clin Gastroenterol Hepatol 2013. [Epub ahead of print].
21. Truelove SC, Witts LJ. Cortisone in ulcerative colitis; final report on a therapeutic trial. Br Med J 1955;2(4947):1041–8.
22. Truelove SC, Richards WC. Biopsy studies in ulcerative colitis. Br Med J 1956; 1(4979):1315–8.
23. Baron JH, Connell AM, Lennard-Jones JE. Variation between observers in describing mucosal appearances in proctocolitis. Br Med J 1964;1:89–92.
24. Powell-Tuck J, Day DW, Buckell NA, et al. Correlations between defined sigmoidoscopic appearances and other measures of disease activity in ulcerative colitis. Dig Dis Sci 1982;27(6):533–7.
25. Sutherland LR, Martin F, Greer S, et al. 5-Aminosalicylic acid enema in the treatment of distal ulcerative colitis, proctosigmoiditis, and proctitis. Gastroenterology 1987;92(6):1894–8.
26. Schroeder KW, Tremaine WJ, Ilstrup DM. Coated oral 5-aminosalicylic acid therapy for mildly to moderately active ulcerative colitis. A randomized study. N Engl J Med 1987;317(26):1625–9.
27. Rachmilewitz D. Coated mesalazine (5-aminosalicylic acid) versus sulphasalazine in the treatment of active ulcerative colitis: a randomised trial. BMJ 1989; 298(6666):82–6.
28. Feagan BG, Greenberg GR, Wild G, et al. Treatment of ulcerative colitis with a humanized antibody to the alpha4beta7 integrin. N Engl J Med 2005;352(24): 2499–507.
29. Naganuma M, Ichikawa H, Inoue N, et al. Novel endoscopic activity index is useful for choosing treatment in severe active ulcerative colitis patients. J Gastroenterol 2010;45(9):936–43.
30. Matts SG. The value of rectal biopsy in the diagnosis of ulcerative colitis. Q J Med 1961;30:393–407.
31. Travis SP, Schnell D, Krzeski P, et al. Developing an instrument to assess the endoscopic severity of ulcerative colitis: the ulcerative colitis endoscopic index of severity (UCEIS). Gut 2012;61(4):535–42.

32. Travis SP, Schnell D, Krzeski P, et al. Reliability and initial validation of the ulcerative colitis endoscopic index of severity. Gastroenterology 2013;145(5):987–95.

33. Travis SP, Higgins PD, Orchard T, et al. Review article: defining remission in ulcerative colitis. Aliment Pharmacol Ther 2011;34(2):113–24.

34. D'Haens G, Feagan B, Colombel JF, et al. Challenges to the design, execution, and analysis of randomized controlled trials for inflammatory bowel disease. Gastroenterology 2012;143(6):1461–9.

35. Kamm MA, Sandborn WJ, Gassull M, et al. Once-daily, high-concentration MMX mesalamine in active ulcerative colitis. Gastroenterology 2007;132(1):66–75.

36. Rutgeerts P, Sandborn WJ, Feagan BG, et al. Infliximab for induction and maintenance therapy for ulcerative colitis. N Engl J Med 2005;353(23):2462–76.

37. Thia KT, Loftus EV, Pardi DS, et al. Measurement of disease activity in ulcerative colitis: interobserver agreement and predictors of severity. Inflamm Bowel Dis 2011;17(6):1257–64.

38. Pola S, Feagan BG, Fahmy M, et al. Observer agreement and construct validity in central endoscopic assessment of disease activity in ulcerative colitis. Gastroenterology 2013;144(5):S-763.

39. Corte CJ, Fernandopulle AN, Catuneanu A, et al. Correlation between the ulcerative colitis endoscopic index of severity (UCEIS) and outcomes in acute severe ulcerative colitis. Gastroenterology 2013;144(5):S-102.

40. Mary JY, Modigliani R. Development and validation of an endoscopic index of the severity for Crohn's disease: a prospective multicentre study. Groupe d'Etudes Thérapeutiques des Affections Inflammatoires du Tube Digestif (GETAID). Gut 1989;30(7):983–9.

41. Daperno M, D'Haens G, Van Assche G, et al. Development and validation of a new, simplified endoscopic activity score for Crohn's disease: the SES-CD. Gastrointest Endosc 2004;60(4):505–12.

42. Rutgeerts P, Geboes K, Vantrappen G, et al. Predictability of the postoperative course of Crohn's disease. Gastroenterology 1990;99(4):956–63.

43. Hébuterne X, Lémann M, Bouhnik Y, et al. Endoscopic improvement of mucosal lesions in patients with moderate to severe ileocolonic Crohn's disease following treatment with certolizumab pegol. Gut 2013;62(2):201–8.

44. Rutgeerts P, Geboes K, Vantrappen G, et al. Natural history of recurrent Crohn's disease at the ileocolonic anastomosis after curative surgery. Gut 1984;25(6):665–72.

45. De Cruz P, Kamm MA, Hamilton AL, et al. Optimising post-operative Crohn's disease management: best drug therapy alone versus colonoscopic monitoring with treatment step-up. The POCER study. Gastroenterology 2013;144(5):S-164.

Quality Bowel Preparation for Surveillance Colonoscopy in Patients with Inflammatory Bowel Disease Is a Must

CrossMark

Andrew Nett, MD[a], Fernando Velayos, MD, MPH[a],
Kenneth McQuaid, MD, FASGE[b],*

KEYWORDS

- Bowel preparation • Inflammatory bowel disease • Dysplasia surveillance

KEY POINTS

- Split-dose bowel regimens should be used in patients without increased risk for gastric retention or aspiration.
- Excessive prepreparation dietary restriction may worsen patient tolerability and preparation quality.
- Patient education enhances patient compliance and bowel preparation quality.
- Suboptimal bowel preparation may negatively affect dysplasia detection.

INTRODUCTION

Patients with inflammatory bowel disease (IBD) are at increased risk of developing colorectal cancer. Compared with sporadic cases, IBD-related colorectal cancers occur at a younger age,[1] are more likely multifocal or synchronous,[2,3] and have a more aggressive phenotype with worsened mortality.[3,4] In light of the increased risk of colorectal cancer, regular colonoscopy is advised every 1 to 3 years in patients for surveillance of colorectal neoplasia. Candidates for surveillance are those with disease duration of 8 years or more who have either ulcerative colitis extending beyond the rectum or Crohn's disease involving one-third or more of the colon. Strong, albeit indirect, data[5–8] suggest a benefit to colonoscopic surveillance. It is therefore recommended by numerous professional guidelines[9–12] and has become widely adopted in standard practice.

The authors have no conflict of interests to disclose.
[a] Department of Medicine, University of California, San Francisco, 513 Parnassus Avenue, Room S-357, San Francisco, CA 94143, USA; [b] Department of Medicine, San Francisco VA Medical Center, University of California, San Francisco, 4150 Clement Street, Room 111-B, San Francisco, CA 94121, USA
* Corresponding author.
E-mail address: krmcq@comcast.net

Gastrointest Endoscopy Clin N Am 24 (2014) 379–392
http://dx.doi.org/10.1016/j.giec.2014.03.004
1052-5157/14/$ – see front matter Published by Elsevier Inc.

IMPORTANCE OF BOWEL PREPARATION

The purpose of surveillance colonoscopy in IBD is to detect neoplasia (ie, cancer or precancerous dysplasia). Until recently, common surveillance technique has entailed a combination of targeted and random biopsies. All visible lesions receive targeted biopsy or resection (via polypectomy or endoscopic mucosal resection) to determine the histology and, most especially, the presence of dysplasia or cancer. In addition, by US guidelines, at least 33 additional random biopsies are taken throughout the colon to detect the presence of flat, endoscopically invisible dysplasia. However, with the advent of enhanced endoscopic imaging, it is increasingly recognized that most IBD-related dysplasia is visible with careful mucosal inspection using high-definition endoscopes and chromoendoscopy. In chromoendoscopy, a solution containing dilute indigo carmine or methylene blue is applied to the mucosal surface via the forward wash jet or biopsy channel to enhance lesion detection (**Fig. 1**). Augmented lesion recognition via chromoendoscopy may supplant the need for random biopsy. A meta-analysis by Soetikno and colleagues[13] confirmed that chromoendoscopy with targeted biopsies of visualized lesions resulted in increased dysplasia detection rates compared with standard white light endoscopy and random biopsies. Several guidelines[12,14,15] now endorse the routine use of chromoendoscopy and question any incremental benefit of random biopsies to detect invisible dysplasia.

This shift in surveillance practice toward targeted lesion biopsy (with endoscopic resection if possible) relies on the premise that even subtle dysplastic lesions are detectable with enhanced imaging techniques. Consequently, a meticulous bowel preparation is critical to facilitate detection of nonpolypoid (flat, slightly raised, or

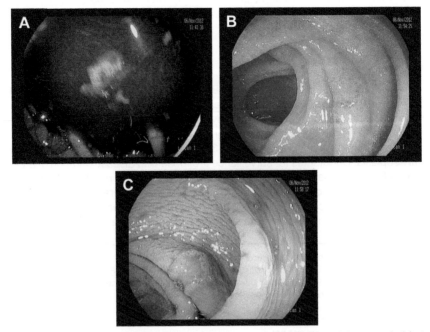

Fig. 1. (*A*) Poor bowel preparation preventing mucosal visualization. (*B*) Concealed lesion shown after irrigation and suctioning. (*C*) Lesion visualization enhanced by chromoendoscopy dye application. (*Courtesy of* Silvia Sanduleanu, MD, PhD, Maastricht University, Maastricht, The Netherlands.)

depressed) lesions, which may be extremely obscure and easily hidden by residual fecal matter, succus, or purgative solution (**Fig. 2**). Although studies have not specifically examined the impact of inadequate bowel preparation on IBD surveillance outcomes, there is clear evidence in the general population that inadequate preparation negatively affects outcomes of screening or surveillance colonoscopy and increases resource use. Bowel preparation is inadequate in nearly 1 of 4 colonoscopies.[16,17] Furthermore, suboptimal preparation results in aborted or incomplete examinations in up to 7% of cases and leads to early recall for surveillance in 12.5% to 20% of cases.[18] Suboptimal preparation also negatively affects colonoscopy efficiency, being associated with prolonged cecal intubation times, decreased cecal intubation rates, increased withdrawal time, and increased perceived procedural difficulty.[19]

Most importantly, suboptimal bowel preparation is associated with lower polyp detection rates, affecting detection of flat (nonpolypoid) lesions[20] and small polyps,[16] as well as large polyps (>10 mm).[19] Among patients undergoing colonoscopy less than 3 years after a previous examination with suboptimal bowel preparation, 42% of all adenomas and 27% of advanced adenomas were found only after the repeat examination. Among examinations performed within 1 year of the initial suboptimal examination, the advanced adenoma miss rate was 36%, suggesting these lesions were truly missed.[17] In another series of 133 patients undergoing repeat colonoscopy after previous suboptimal preparation, missed adenomas were found in 34%. A high-risk state was present in 18% of patients (ie, the presence of ≥3 adenomas, 1 adenoma >1 cm, or adenomas with high-grade dysplasia or villous features).[21] Similarly, Sagi and colleagues[22] reported that among patients undergoing early examination as a result of initial suboptimal bowel preparation, 6.5% had high-risk adenomas and 1.9% had high-grade dysplasia or cancer.

It is evident from the literature that inadequate preparation negatively affects the performance of colonoscopy in patients who do not have IBD. Although not directly

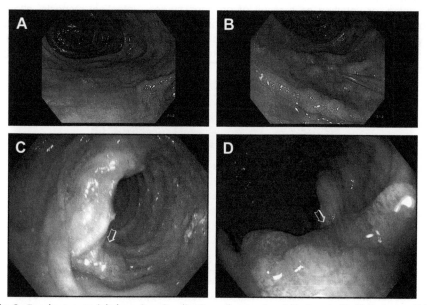

Fig. 2. Feculent material obscuring visualization of nonpolypoid lesions in (*A, B*) Crohn's colitis and (*C, D*) ulcerative colitis. (*Courtesy of* Roy Soetikno, MD, Veterans Affairs, Palo Alto, CA.)

studied in patients with IBD undergoing surveillance, a meticulous bowel preparation facilitates detection of IBD-related neoplasia, particularly nonpolypoid lesions. Flat dysplasia detection in patients with IBD has been shown to be directly correlated with procedure duration.[23] Although the underlying reason for this association is unproven, prolonged withdrawal may reflect careful mucosal inspection. Poor preparation requiring lengthy irrigation may lessen total inspection time.

An impeccable bowel preparation is especially important for chromoendoscopy surveillance techniques.[24] Personal and anecdotal shared experiences affirm the negative impact of suboptimal bowel preparation on the efficient application of chromoendoscopy. The admixture of chromoendoscopy dye with retained colonic soilage results in flocculent, green debris, which can obscure subtle lesions and require copious irrigation to achieve an acceptable mucosal inspection (**Fig. 3**).

PREDICTORS OF SUBOPTIMAL BOWEL PREPARATION

In patients without IBD, the known predictors of poor bowel preparation include advanced age, male gender, diabetes, obesity, multiple comorbidities, tricyclic antidepressant or opiate use, inpatient status, immobility, and lower education level.[25–27] Most studies examining risk factors for poor colonic preparation do not assess the impact of IBD.[25] When specifically evaluated, no significant difference in bowel preparation quality was detected between patients with IBD and those who did not have IBD, as rated by the Boston Bowel Preparation Scale. Nor did an association exist between IBD disease activity and preparation quality.[28] Thus, there is no definitive proof that patients with IBD have an increased likelihood of inadequate bowel preparation.

Notwithstanding this limited published experience, personal and anecdotal experience suggests increased difficulty with bowel preparation in some patients with IBD. Bowel preparation is of poorer quality in patients with previous colonic resections,[29,30] including patients with and without IBD, possibly because of disturbances in intestinal motility. Furthermore, some patients with IBD have increased nausea, bloating, cramping, or vomiting as a result of previous surgery, intestinal stenosis, altered motility, anxiety, or heightened visceral sensitivity. In a case control study by Bessissow and colleagues,[28] patients with IBD did not experience increased levels of nausea or pain during bowel preparation overall, but patients with active Crohn's disease did

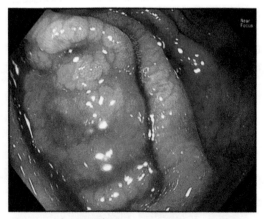

Fig. 3. Poor preparation interferes with chromoendoscopy. Admixture of stool, dye, and mucus interferes with mucosal visualization. (*Courtesy of* Roy Soetikno, MD, Veterans Affairs, Palo Alto, CA.)

experience higher levels of abdominal pain. A higher level of anxiety was also associated with increased symptoms during bowel preparation, and patients with IBD experience significantly more embarrassment and burden (defined as feelings of worry, hardship, or distress) during preparation when compared with patients undergoing colonoscopy for other indications.[31] Furthermore, in a study assessing factors affecting adherence with surveillance recommendations,[32] patients with IBD most commonly cited difficulty with bowel preparation as the most important reason for failed compliance. Thus, although limited clinical studies do not convincingly show a higher incidence of suboptimal bowel preparations in patients with IBD, ample data confirm a reduced tolerance of the bowel preparation, which may negatively affect bowel preparation quality and compliance with surveillance protocols.

OPTIMIZATION OF BOWEL PREPARATION
Bowel Preparation in Patients with Active Inflammation

Optimization of the preparation protocol helps to promote thorough colonic preparation and maximize surveillance benefit. The best strategy for preparation in patients with IBD may vary depending on the indication for colonoscopy. In patients with active symptoms undergoing endoscopy to assess the activity and extent of disease, considerations include the potential complications of aggressive bowel preparation in the context of active inflammation. For example, partial obstruction caused by fixed or inflammatory strictures, delayed gastric emptying (medication or disease-related), hospitalization status, and urgency of the examination may all affect the bowel preparation regimen, including the choice of purgative, and the frequency, rate, and mode of purgative delivery. Concern for partial or high-grade obstruction may favor the use of small-volume, oral solutions supplemented by intravenous hydration or the use of a slow oral trickle preparation delivered over longer periods rather than more rapid administration of large-volume solutions. Furthermore, use of split-dosing regimens (which include same-day purgative administration 4–6 hours before endoscopy) may be contraindicated in the setting of mechanically delayed intestinal transit because of higher aspiration risk. Patients with severe active colitis and diarrhea may require only minimal laxative administration to achieve adequate preparation for disease staging because of rapid transit, the absence of solid fecal matter, and decreased adherence of liquid stool to the intestinal wall. British National Health Service guidelines[33] designate severe acute active inflammation as an absolute contraindication to oral preparation administration. Thus, in patients with active disease, safety factors and disease-related symptoms make a pristine colon a less rigid goal of bowel preparation.

Bowel Preparation in Patients Undergoing Surveillance

In contrast, a meticulous bowel preparation is important in patients undergoing routine, elective colonoscopy for dysplasia surveillance. Whenever possible, the disease should be in remission at the time of surveillance colonoscopy, because active inflammation interferes with visual detection of nonpolypoid dysplasia and causes cytologic changes, which can be difficult to distinguish from true dysplasia. Complications of active inflammation therefore are of lesser concern, and preparation decisions focus on achieving maximum bowel cleanliness.

The best preparation regimen consists of an appropriate preprocedure diet, a suitable choice of laxative agent, and an optimal dosing of laxative administration. It is vitally important that physicians and nursing staff educate patients about the importance of the bowel preparation, carefully reviewing recommended dietary restrictions and counseling strict adherence to bowel preparation instructions. The remainder of this article emphasizes recommended, established preparation techniques for the purpose of nonurgent surveillance in patients with controlled disease.

Prepreparation dietary restriction

There are several uncertainties regarding the best preprocedure diet. In the days leading up to colonoscopy, many centers advise patients to avoid foods containing small seeds (eg, tomatoes and cucumbers) based on concern that colonoscopy efficiency can be diminished by clogging of the endoscope suction channel. This problem does arise, especially among patients with diverticulosis, although there is no literature studying the degree of encumbrance. Other routine advice includes several days of avoidance of high-fiber food or supplements, especially iron-containing supplements, which cause blackening of stool with increased adhesion of remnant stool to the bowel wall.

On the day preceding colonoscopy, patients are routinely instructed to consume only clear liquids. Many centers also advise patients to forego red-colored food products such as red gelatin, red juices, or red soft drinks to avoid confusion regarding the presence of possible blood. However, the rate of false alarm caused by these products has not been studied, and anecdotal experience suggests that their consumption is unlikely to create diagnostic uncertainty with the use of proven high-quality bowel preparation regimens.

Several recent studies have suggested that rigid adherence to a clear liquid diet on the day preceding the procedure may also be unnecessary (**Table 1**). Dietary liberalization may allow for improved tolerance and better adherence without compromise of bowel preparation quality.[34] In some studies, a less restrictive diet increases bowel preparation quality.[35–37]

Frequency and timing of bowel laxative preparations: importance of split regimens

The most critical component of bowel preparation is the use of an appropriate laxative regimen. Regardless of the type of laxative prescribed (**Table 2**), there is overwhelming evidence from randomized controlled trials supporting of the use of split-dosing regimens. In these regimens, partial laxative administration occurs on the evening before colonoscopy, with the remainder administered within 2 to 6 hours before colonoscopy. A meta-analysis performed by Kilgore and colleagues[38] of 5 randomized controlled trials showed that, compared with single, full-dose administration of 4 L polyethylene glycol (PEG) solution on the evening before the procedure, the administration of split-dose PEG preparations (2 L the evening before the procedure and 2 L completed by 2 hours before the procedure) resulted in a higher likelihood of satisfactory bowel preparations (odds ratio [OR] 3.7; 95% confidence interval [CI] 2.79–4.41), an increased willingness to repeat the same preparation, and decreased nausea. Another systematic review by Enestvedt and colleagues[39] of 9 trials comparing 4 L split-dose PEG preparations with various other bowel preparation regimens (4 L single dose or smaller volume split dose) confirmed a significantly higher likelihood of excellent or good bowel preparation with the 4 L split-dose regimen (OR 3.46; 95% CI 2.45–4.89). No difference existed between the 4-L split-dose PEG formulations and alternative preparations in regards to patient compliance, willingness to repeat preparation, overall experience, or symptoms of abdominal cramping, nausea, or sleep disturbance. A recent study has confirmed that use of a split-dose 3-L PEG/ascorbic acid preparation (2 L PM, 1 L AM) not only improved bowel preparation quality but also was associated with increased adenoma detection rates.[40] Based on the proven superiority of split-dose bowel regimens over single-dose regimens, professional guidelines[41,42] now recommend use of split-dose preparation.

Table 1
Effect of less restrictive prepreparation diet on bowel preparation quality and tolerability

Study	N	Prepreparation Diet			Bowel Preparation	Dosing	Bowel Preparation Quality	Better Patient Tolerability
		Diets Compared	Duration of Dietary Liberalization[a]					
Soweid et al,[35] 2010	200	Fiber free vs clear liquid	Entire day		4 L PEG-ELS	Single	Fiber free > clear liquid	Fiber free
Park et al,[36] 2009	214	Low residue vs clear liquid	Entire day		4 L PEG-ELS	Single	Low residue > clear liquid	Low residue
Melicharkova et al, 2013	213	Low residue vs clear liquid	Breakfast		Na picosulfate/ magnesium citrate	Single	No difference	Low residue
Sipe et al,[34] 2013	196	Low residue vs clear liquid	Breakfast + lunch + snack		Sulfate solution	Split	No difference	Low residue
Jung et al,[56] 2013	801	Regular[b] vs clear liquid	Entire day		4 L PEG-ELS	Single	No difference	No difference

[a] Portion of the day before colonoscopy in which 1 group in comparative trial was allowed a diet less restrictive than clear liquids.
[b] Although groups were assigned to either regular intake or a clear liquid diet on the day before colonoscopy, patients in both groups were advised to avoid high-fiber foods in the 3 days before colonoscopy.[56]

Table 2
Laxative options for bowel preparation

Type	Total Volume	Product Name	FDA-Approved Dosing	Split Dosing Reported?
Isosmotic				
Standard PEG-ELS	4 L	GoLytely Colyte Generic	Single day	Yes
Sulfate-free PEG-ELS	4 L	NuLytely TriLyte	Single day	Yes
Sulfate-free PEG-ELS + preceding bisacodyl	2 L	HalfLytely	Single day	No
PEG-ELS with ascorbate	3 L	MoviPrep	Single day or split	Yes
Gatorade + Miralax 238 g	2 L	Gatorade + Miralax	Not FDA approved	Yes
Hyperosmotic				
Sodium/potassium/magnesium sulfate and PEG-ELS	3.5 L	Suclear	Single day or split	Yes
Sulfate solution (sodium sulfate, potassium sulfate, magnesium sulfate)	3 L	Suprep	Split	Yes
Sodium picosulfate, magnesium oxide, citrate	2.2 L	Prepopik	Single day or split	Yes
Sodium phosphate tablets	2 L	OsmoPrep	Split	Yes

Abbreviations: ELS, electrolyte lavage solution; FDA, US Food and Drug Administration; PEG, polyethylene glycol.

Morning consumption of laxative as part of a split-dose regimen creates 2 concerns. First, patients may be resistant to waking early to complete the laxative. Despite this pragmatic consideration, patients do generally accept and comply with split dosing. Unger and colleagues[43] reported 78% compliance with a split dose in patients receiving early morning colonoscopy. Several studies[44,45] have also shown that patients better tolerate split-dosing preparations.

The second concern pertains to the safety of split-dosing administration. Specifically, ingestion of the second dose of a bowel laxative within 2 to 6 hours of colonoscopy might increase the risk for aspiration during sedation (moderate, deep, or general anesthesia). Updated guidelines from the American Society of Anesthesiologists[46] state that patients need to abstain from clear liquids for only 2 hours before receiving sedation. Nonetheless, some anesthesiologists question the clinical and safety equivalency of PEG solutions to other clear liquids. In addressing these concerns, despite widespread use of PEG solutions for almost 30 years in millions of patients, there are only rare (<12), isolated reports of fatal, aspiration-induced chemical pneumonitis after administration of a PEG solution (most commonly occurring with nasogastric administration in adults or children with altered mental status). Furthermore, a 2010 study[47] showed no difference in residual gastric volume in patients taking a split-dose bowel preparation (19.7 mL) versus a single-dose evening preparation (20.2 mL).

Therefore, based on their proven superiority, split-dose bowel regimens should be recommended for most patients with IBD undergoing surveillance whose disease is in remission or well controlled. Caution is advised in patients with partial bowel obstruction, gastroparesis, or known delayed intestinal motility, because these patients are at increased risk for gastric retention and aspiration. In these instances, a 6-hour window is recommended between completion of the laxative ingestion and initiation of sedation.

Available preparation formulations: how to choose

Several laxative formulations are available for preparation before colonoscopy. Randomized controlled trials comparing these agents are limited, and none has proven superiority. However, for all available agents, a split-dose regimen generally is preferred to single-dose regimens.

Laxative options may be subsumed under 2 broad categories: PEG solutions and low-volume, hyperosmolar solutions (see **Table 2**). Several PEG solutions are available, including full-volume (4 L) balanced, isosmotic formulations (standard or sulfate-free) and a reduced volume (3 L) formulation, which contains ascorbate. In general, split dosing of PEG solutions achieves good or excellent bowel preparation quality in 75% to 95% of patients compared with less than 60% with single-dose administration. Although some endoscopy centers recommend the use of a split-dose administration of a 2-L homemade solution of Gatorade plus PEG-3350 (Miralax), a meta-analysis has found this regimen to be inferior to standard, split-dose 4-L PEG solutions.[39]

Two low-volume hyperosmolar solutions that do not contain PEG are available, but both must be taken with sufficient amounts of water to promote adequate cleansing. These solutions include a sulfate solution (Suprep, 3 L, including water) and a magnesium citrate/picosulfate solution (Prepopik, 2.2 L, including water). Because these hyperosmolar solutions may cause dehydration and electrolyte shifts, they should be used with caution in patients with significant renal or cardiac disease or in patients unable or unlikely to comply with instructions. There are no controlled trials comparing split dosing of low-volume, hyperosmolar solutions and split dosing of standard large-volume 4-L PEG solutions, and hence, it is unknown whether these low-volume options provide comparable outcomes. A trial[48] comparing split dosing of a low-volume sulfate-based preparation with split dosing of a low-volume (2 L) PEG solution containing ascorbic acid (MoviPrep) yielded a comparable proportion of good or excellent preparations.

Most recently, another preparation (Suclear) has become available, in which a sulfate solution (1 L, including water) is administered the evening before the procedure, and balanced PEG solution (2 L) is administered 4 hours before the procedure. In a controlled trial, split dosing of the sulfate/PEG formulation achieved a similar level of acceptable bowel preparation as split dosing of a low-volume (2 L) PEG/ascorbic acid solution.[49] Phosphate-based preparations (tablets and solutions) are still available but have significant potential for adverse consequences. These preparations can induce mucosal ulcerations that mimic IBD, confusing disease diagnosis and staging. More importantly, several reported cases of severe hyperphosphatemia have occurred (some complicated by mortality) as well as cases of acute phosphate nephropathy. Because of safety concerns as well as the availability of numerous alternative preparation options, phosphate-based solutions should be avoided.[50]

No studies have compared specific preparation types in patients with IBD. Thus, physicians and endoscopy centers may favor particular agents based on personal experience, reported patient satisfaction, and cost considerations. Based on the extensive body of literature supporting their efficacy and safety, bowel regimens with a split-dose of a full-volume (4 L) balanced PEG solution may be recommended for most patients. The European Society of Gastrointestinal Endoscopy[51] specifically recommends use of a PEG formulation in patients with IBD, because alternative

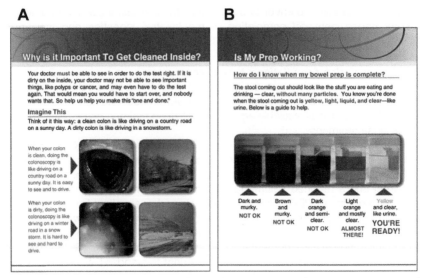

Fig. 4. Sample images from educational pamphlet shown to enhance preparation quality. (*From* Spiegel BM, Talley J, Shekelle P, et al. Development and validation of a novel patient educational booklet to enhance colonoscopy preparation. Am J Gastroenterol 2011;106(5): 875–83; with permission.)

formulations can cause mucosal damage. However, as noted earlier, patients with IBD commonly cite difficulty with bowel preparation as a reason for nonadherence to a surveillance program. Thus, in patients with previous intolerance of large-volume preparations or in whom intolerance is anticipated because of heightened anxiety, low-volume alternatives should be considered to improve compliance, provided there are no contraindications to these agents (renal, cardiac, or liver disease).

Patient Education

Patient education may enhance bowel preparation quality by promoting adherence to the preparation regimen. Rosenfeld and colleagues[52] showed that inpatients receiving a 5-minute educational talk regarding the reason for bowel preparation and the importance of preparation completion had improved preparation quality. Likewise, in a controlled trial of 436 patients, the patients randomized to receive an educational booklet had improved satisfactory bowel preparation quality (76%) compared with those not receiving a booklet (46%).[53] Clear visual references show patients specific end points of colonic preparation (**Fig. 4**). Other studies also have confirmed the usefulness of cartoon visual aids[54] and educational pamphlets[55] in promoting improved bowel preparation quality.

SUMMARY

IBD surveillance mandates scrupulous bowel preparation to optimize detection of nonpolypoid dysplasia. Split-dose administration of a PEG-based regimen is recommended in patients without contraindications. Some patients with IBD may have reduced tolerance of bowel preparation. Low-volume preparations should be considered in patients with known stenosis, dysmotility, anxiety, active disease, or previous preparation intolerance to promote adherence to surveillance protocols. Avoidance of unnecessary dietary restriction and provision of thorough patient education also enhance patient tolerance and compliance.

REFERENCES

1. Delaunoit T, Limburg PJ, Goldberg RM, et al. Colorectal cancer prognosis among patients with inflammatory bowel disease. Clin Gastroenterol Hepatol 2006;4(3):335–42.
2. Greenstein AJ, Slater G, Heimann TM, et al. A comparison of multiple synchronous colorectal cancer in ulcerative colitis, familial polyposis coli, and de novo cancer. Ann Surg 1986;203(2):123–8.
3. Watanabe T, Konishi T, Kishimoto J, et al. Ulcerative colitis-associated colorectal cancer shows a poorer survival than sporadic colorectal cancer: a nationwide Japanese study. Inflamm Bowel Dis 2011;17(3):802–8.
4. Ording AG, Horvath-Puho E, Erichsen R, et al. Five-year mortality in colorectal cancer patients with ulcerative colitis or Crohn's disease: a nationwide population-based cohort study. Inflamm Bowel Dis 2013;19(4):800–5.
5. Wang YR, Cangemi JR, Loftus EV Jr, et al. Rate of early/missed colorectal cancers after colonoscopy in older patients with or without inflammatory bowel disease in the United States. Am J Gastroenterol 2013;108(3):444–9.
6. Lutgens MW, Oldenburg B, Siersema PD, et al. Colonoscopic surveillance improves survival after colorectal cancer diagnosis in inflammatory bowel disease. Br J Cancer 2009;101(10):1671–5.
7. Karlen P, Kornfeld D, Brostrom O, et al. Is colonoscopic surveillance reducing colorectal cancer mortality in ulcerative colitis? A population based case control study. Gut 1998;42(5):711–4.
8. Collins PD. Strategies for detecting colon cancer and dysplasia in patients with inflammatory bowel disease. Inflamm Bowel Dis 2013;19(4):860–3.
9. Farraye FA, Odze RD, Eaden J, et al. AGA medical position statement on the diagnosis and management of colorectal neoplasia in inflammatory bowel disease. Gastroenterology 2010;138(2):738–45.
10. Kornbluth A, Sachar DB, Practice Parameters Committee of the American College of Gastroenterology. Ulcerative colitis practice guidelines in adults: American College of Gastroenterology, Practice Parameters Committee. Am J Gastroenterol 2010;105(3):501–23 [quiz: 524].
11. Leighton JA, Shen B, Baron TH, et al. ASGE guideline: endoscopy in the diagnosis and treatment of inflammatory bowel disease. Gastrointest Endosc 2006;63(4):558–65.
12. Cairns SR, Scholefield JH, Steele RJ, et al. Guidelines for colorectal cancer screening and surveillance in moderate and high risk groups (update from 2002). Gut 2010;59(5):666–89.
13. Soetikno R, Subramanian V, Kaltenbach T, et al. The detection of nonpolypoid (flat and depressed) colorectal neoplasms in patients with inflammatory bowel disease. Gastroenterology 2013;144(7):1349–52, 1352.e1–6.
14. Clinical practice guidelines for surveillance colonoscopy–in adenoma follow-up; following curative resection of colorectal cancer; and for cancer surveillance in inflammatory bowel disease. Cancer Council Australia (December 2011).
15. Van Assche G, Dignass A, Bokemeyer B, et al. Second European evidence-based consensus on the diagnosis and management of ulcerative colitis part 3: special situations. J Crohns Colitis 2013;7(1):1–33.

16. Harewood GC, Sharma VK, de Garmo P. Impact of colonoscopy preparation quality on detection of suspected colonic neoplasia. Gastrointest Endosc 2003;58(1):76–9.
17. Lebwohl B, Kastrinos F, Glick M, et al. The impact of suboptimal bowel preparation on adenoma miss rates and the factors associated with early repeat colonoscopy. Gastrointest Endosc 2011;73(6):1207–14.
18. Rex DK, Imperiale TF, Latinovich DR, et al. Impact of bowel preparation on efficiency and cost of colonoscopy. Am J Gastroenterol 2002;97(7):1696–700.
19. Froehlich F, Wietlisbach V, Gonvers JJ, et al. Impact of colonic cleansing on quality and diagnostic yield of colonoscopy: The European Panel of Appropriateness of Gastrointestinal Endoscopy European multicenter study. Gastrointest Endosc 2005;61(3):378–84.
20. Parra-Blanco A, Nicolas-Perez D, Gimeno-Garcia A, et al. The timing of bowel preparation before colonoscopy determines the quality of cleansing, and is a significant factor contributing to the detection of flat lesions: a randomized study. World J Gastroenterol 2006;12(38):6161–6.
21. Chokshi RV, Hovis CE, Hollander T, et al. Prevalence of missed adenomas in patients with inadequate bowel preparation on screening colonoscopy. Gastrointest Endosc 2012;75(6):1197–203.
22. Sagi SV, Guturu P, Gottumukkala RS. Missed adenomas in patients with inadequate bowel preparation. Gastrointest Endosc 2012;76(3):705.
23. Toruner M, Harewood GC, Loftus EV Jr, et al. Endoscopic factors in the diagnosis of colorectal dysplasia in chronic inflammatory bowel disease. Inflamm Bowel Dis 2005;11(5):428–34.
24. Kiesslich R, Neurath MF. Surveillance colonoscopy in ulcerative colitis: magnifying chromoendoscopy in the spotlight. Gut 2004;53(2):165–7.
25. Romero RV, Mahadeva S. Factors influencing quality of bowel preparation for colonoscopy. World J Gastrointest Endosc 2013;5(2):39–46.
26. Nguyen DL, Wieland M. Risk factors predictive of poor quality preparation during average risk colonoscopy screening: the importance of health literacy. J Gastrointestin Liver Dis 2010;19(4):369–72.
27. Chan WK, Saravanan A, Manikam J, et al. Appointment waiting times and education level influence the quality of bowel preparation in adult patients undergoing colonoscopy. BMC Gastroenterol 2011;11:86.
28. Bessissow T, Van Keerberghen CA, Van Oudenhove L, et al. Anxiety is associated with impaired tolerance of colonoscopy preparation in inflammatory bowel disease and controls. J Crohns Colitis 2013;7(11):e580–7.
29. Lim SW, Seo YW, Sinn DH, et al. Impact of previous gastric or colonic resection on polyethylene glycol bowel preparation for colonoscopy. Surg Endosc 2012; 26(6):1554–9.
30. Chung YW, Han DS, Park KH, et al. Patient factors predictive of inadequate bowel preparation using polyethylene glycol: a prospective study in Korea. J Clin Gastroenterol 2009;43(5):448–52.
31. Denters MJ, Schreuder M, Depla AC, et al. Patients' perception of colonoscopy: patients with inflammatory bowel disease and irritable bowel syndrome experience the largest burden. Eur J Gastroenterol Hepatol 2013;25(8):964–72.
32. Friedman S, Cheifetz AS, Farraye FA, et al. Factors that affect adherence to surveillance colonoscopy in patients with inflammatory bowel disease. Inflamm Bowel Dis 2013;19(3):534–9.
33. Connor A, Tolan D, Hughes S, et al. Consensus guidelines for the safe prescription and administration of oral bowel-cleansing agents. Gut 2012;61(11):1525–32.

34. Sipe BW, Fischer M, Baluyut AR, et al. A low-residue diet improved patient satisfaction with split-dose oral sulfate solution without impairing colonic preparation. Gastrointest Endosc 2013;77(6):932–6.

35. Soweid AM, Kobeissy AA, Jamali FR, et al. A randomized single-blind trial of standard diet versus fiber-free diet with polyethylene glycol electrolyte solution for colonoscopy preparation. Endoscopy 2010;42(8):633–8.

36. Park DI, Park SH, Lee SK, et al. Efficacy of prepackaged, low residual test meals with 4L polyethylene glycol versus a clear liquid diet with 4L polyethylene glycol bowel preparation: a randomized trial. J Gastroenterol Hepatol 2009;24(6): 988–91.

37. Delegge M, Kaplan R. Efficacy of bowel preparation with the use of a prepackaged, low fibre diet with a low sodium, magnesium citrate cathartic vs. a clear liquid diet with a standard sodium phosphate cathartic. Aliment Pharmacol Ther 2005;21(12):1491–5.

38. Kilgore TW, Abdinoor AA, Szary NM, et al. Bowel preparation with split-dose polyethylene glycol before colonoscopy: a meta-analysis of randomized controlled trials. Gastrointest Endosc 2011;73(6):1240–5.

39. Enestvedt BK, Tofani C, Laine LA, et al. 4-liter split-dose polyethylene glycol is superior to other bowel preparations, based on systematic review and meta-analysis. Clin Gastroenterol Hepatol 2012;10(11):1225–31.

40. Gurudu SR, Ramirez FC, Harrison ME, et al. Increased adenoma detection rate with system-wide implementation of a split-dose preparation for colonoscopy. Gastrointest Endosc 2012;76(3):603–8.e1.

41. Rex DK, Johnson DA, Anderson JC, et al. American College of Gastroenterology guidelines for colorectal cancer screening 2009 [corrected]. Am J Gastroenterol 2009;104(3):739–50.

42. Wexner SD, Beck DE, Baron TH, et al. A consensus document on bowel preparation before colonoscopy: prepared by a task force from the American Society of Colon and Rectal Surgeons (ASCRS), the American Society for Gastrointestinal Endoscopy (ASGE), and the Society of American Gastrointestinal and Endoscopic Surgeons (SAGES). Gastrointest Endosc 2006;63(7): 894–909.

43. Unger RZ, Amstutz SP, Seo da H, et al. Willingness to undergo split-dose bowel preparation for colonoscopy and compliance with split-dose instructions. Dig Dis Sci 2010;55(7):2030–4.

44. Khan MA, Piotrowski Z, Brown MD. Patient acceptance, convenience, and efficacy of single-dose versus split-dose colonoscopy bowel preparation. J Clin Gastroenterol 2010;44(4):310–1.

45. Park SS, Sinn DH, Kim YH, et al. Efficacy and tolerability of split-dose magnesium citrate: low-volume (2 liters) polyethylene glycol vs. single- or split-dose polyethylene glycol bowel preparation for morning colonoscopy. Am J Gastroenterol 2010;105(6):1319–26.

46. American Society of Anesthesiologists Committee. Practice guidelines for preoperative fasting and the use of pharmacologic agents to reduce the risk of pulmonary aspiration: application to healthy patients undergoing elective procedures: an updated report by the American Society of Anesthesiologists committee on standards and practice parameters. Anesthesiology 2011; 114(3):495–511.

47. Huffman M, Unger RZ, Thatikonda C, et al. Split-dose bowel preparation for colonoscopy and residual gastric fluid volume: an observational study. Gastrointest Endosc 2010;72(3):516–22.

48. Di Palma JA, Rodriguez R, McGowan J, et al. A randomized clinical study evaluating the safety and efficacy of a new, reduced-volume, oral sulfate colon-cleansing preparation for colonoscopy. Am J Gastroenterol 2009;104(9): 2275–84.

49. Suclear(R) [package insert]. Braintree, MA: Braintree Laboratories; 2013. Available at: http://www.suclearkit.com/collateral/documents/suclear/SUCLEAR-PI-MedGuide-MARCH-2013.pdf. Accessed December 12, 2013.

50. Markowitz GS, Stokes MB, Radhakrishnan J, et al. Acute phosphate nephropathy following oral sodium phosphate bowel purgative: an underrecognized cause of chronic renal failure. J Am Soc Nephrol 2005;16(11):3389–96.

51. Hassan C, Bretthauer M, Kaminski MF, et al. Bowel preparation for colonoscopy: European Society of Gastrointestinal Endoscopy (ESGE) guideline. Endoscopy 2013;45(2):142–50.

52. Rosenfeld G, Krygier D, Enns RA, et al. The impact of patient education on the quality of inpatient bowel preparation for colonoscopy. Can J Gastroenterol 2010;24(9):543–6.

53. Spiegel BM, Talley J, Shekelle P, et al. Development and validation of a novel patient educational booklet to enhance colonoscopy preparation. Am J Gastroenterol 2011;106(5):875–83.

54. Tae JW, Lee JC, Hong SJ, et al. Impact of patient education with cartoon visual aids on the quality of bowel preparation for colonoscopy. Gastrointest Endosc 2012;76(4):804–11.

55. Shaikh AA, Hussain SM, Rahn S, et al. Effect of an educational pamphlet on colon cancer screening: a randomized, prospective trial. Eur J Gastroenterol Hepatol 2010;22(4):444–9.

56. Jung YS, Seok HS, Park DI, et al. A clear liquid diet is not mandatory for polyethylene glycol-based bowel preparation for afternoon colonoscopy in healthy outpatients. Gut Liver 2013;7(6):681–7.

Image-Enhanced Endoscopy Is Critical in the Surveillance of Patients with Colonic IBD

Venkataraman Subramanian, MD, DM, MRCP(UK)[a],*,
Raf Bisschops, MD, PhD[b]

KEYWORDS

- Surveillance • Ulcerative colitis • Crohn's disease • Chromoendoscopy
- Narrow band imaging • Autofluorescence • FICE • iSCAN

KEY POINTS

- Cancer risk in patients with colonic inflammatory bowel disease (IBD) is high and increases over time. Quality and efficacy of surveillance is variable in routine clinical practice.
- Chromoendoscopy (CE) is recommended by most societies as the preferred test for colorectal cancer (CRC) surveillance in patients with colonic IBD. It has been shown unequivocally to improve dysplasia detection on targeted biopsies.
- Narrow band imaging has not shown superior dysplasia detected on targeted biopsies compared with CE or with white light imaging.

INTRODUCTION

Patients with IBD involving the colon have an increased risk for CRC compared with the general population.[1] Cancer in ulcerative colitis (UC) occurs at a younger age and increases with time, approaching 18% after 30 years of disease.[1] This increased risk has prompted both the North American and United Kingdom gastroenterology societies to recommend cancer prevention strategies.[2,3]

Disclosure Statement: V. Subramanian has no relevant disclosure to make; R. Bisschops is supported by a research grant from FWO-Vlaanderen. R. Bisschops received speaker's fees from Olympus, Pentax, and Fujifilm Corporation. Both authors contributed to the conception, drafting, critical revision, and final approval of the article.
[a] Molecular Gastroenterology, Leeds Institute of Biomedical and Clinical Sciences, St James University Hospital, University of Leeds, Leeds LS9 7TF, UK; [b] Department of Gastroenterology, University Hospital Leuven, Herestraat 49, 3000 Leuven, Belgium
* Corresponding author.
E-mail address: v.subramanian@leeds.ac.uk

Surveillance colonoscopies for early detection have been widely adopted to formally evaluate the benefits, risks, and costs of this approach.[4–7] Despite surveillance, interval cancer rates are high in these patients. A 2006 Cochrane review found no clear evidence that surveillance colonoscopy prolongs survival in patients with extensive colitis.[8] In the same year, a 30-year analysis of surveillance practice from St Mark's hospital reported that more than 50% of detected cancers were found to be interval cancers.[4] These data reflect an era when dysplasia was perceived to be invisible and only detected on random biopsies.[9]

In the past decade, endoscopic technology and technique has matured, with parallel evidence showing that the vast majority of dysplasia is visible and can be targeted. The long-term effects of surveillance using these new techniques, such as cancer-free survival, are still unknown. In this review, the authors summarize the existing literature on image-enhanced endoscopic techniques for surveillance of long-standing colonic IBD for the detection of dysplasia. They focus on dye-based chromoendoscopic techniques and present electronic-based image-enhanced endoscopic techniques such as narrow band imaging and autofluorescence endoscopy. Confocal laser endomicroscopy, a lesion characterization technology, is described in detail by Kiesslich and Matsumoto in another article in this issue.

SURVEILLANCE TECHNIQUES
Futility of White Light with Random Biopsy

Random mucosal sampling throughout the colon has historically been the mainstay of IBD surveillance colonoscopy. The technique is tedious, expensive, and time consuming, as it requires multiple biopsies to be taken segmentally throughout the colon and processed in separate jars. It has been estimated that at least 33 biopsies are needed to achieve 90% confidence to detect dysplasia if it is present.[10] The technique is not only inefficient but also inefficacious. The yield from random biopsy in studies on surveillance colonoscopy using high-definition (HD) endoscopes or other image-enhancement techniques is poor. **Table 1** summarizes the dysplasia yield from random biopsies for studies using image-enhanced endoscopic technologies.

The need to adopt image-enhanced techniques with targeted lesion detection is underscored by the low yield and unknown clinical significance from dysplasia found on random biopsies. Van den Broek and colleagues[20] published a retrospective analysis of the yield of dysplasia and clinical significance of dysplasia detected in random biopsies. Of 466 colonoscopies involving 167 patients done in a 10-year period from 1998 to 2008, dysplasia was detected by random biopsy only in 5 colonoscopies involving 4 patients. Only in one of these patients did protocolectomy confirm the presence of advanced neoplasia.

Superiority of Chromoendoscopy with Targeted Biopsy

The British Society of Gastroenterology[21] and the European Crohn's and Colitis organization[22] have specified chromoendoscopy (CE) as the preferred modality for surveillance in patients with colonic IBD. CE refers to the topical application of dyes (indigo carmine[23] or methylene blue[24]) to improve detection and delineation of surface abnormalities by pooling into mucosal crevices. Its application enhances the detection of subtle mucosal abnormalities to improve the yield of surveillance,[16] compared with white light inspection alone. Both indigo carmine and methylene blue have been widely used and shown to be effective. CE was first shown to be useful in the detection of flat adenomas in the sporadic setting and in patients with familial polyposis

Table 1
Yield of dysplasia from random biopsies in prospective endoscopic studies involving surveillance colonoscopy with image-enhanced endoscopy for colonic IBD in the last 10 years

Study Author, Year	Country	Image-Enhanced Modality Used	Number of Patients	Number of Random Biopsies with Dysplasia	Total Number of Random Biopsies	Mean Number of Random Biopsies per Episode of Dysplasia
Kiesslich et al,[11] 2003	Germany	Methylene blue chromoendoscopy	165	2 (in white light arm only)	5098	2549
Matsumoto et al,[12] 2003	Japan	Indigo carmine chromoendoscopy	57	3	702	234
Rutter et al,[13] 2004	United Kingdom	Indigo carmine chromoendoscopy	100	0	2904	—
Kiesslich et al,[14] 2007	Germany	Methylene blue chromoendoscopy	153	2 (in white light arm only)	2854	1427
Dekker et al,[15] 2007	Netherlands	Narrow Band Imaging (first generation)	42	1	1522	1522
Van den Broek et al,[16] 2008	Netherlands	Autofluorescence endoscopy	50	2	1992	996
Marion et al,[17] 2008	USA	Methylene blue chromoendoscopy	102	3	3264	1088
Van den Broek et al,[18] 2011	Netherlands	Narrow Band Imaging (second generation)	48	3	1580	527
Ignjatovic et al,[19] 2012	United Kingdom	Narrow Band Imaging (second generation)	112	1	2707	2707

syndromes[25,26]; during the past decade, studies have also shown CE to augment the visualization of dysplasia in UC.[27,28]

Table 2 lists the published studies comparing pancolonic CE with WLE for detection of dysplasia in colonic IBD. A meta-analysis of the available data in 2011[32] and an updated one in 2013[33] that included 6 studies with 665 patients confirmed the superiority of CE with targeted biopsy to standard WLE with random biopsy. A 6% increase in the yield of dysplasia was noted in the most recent analysis, leading to a number needed to treat of 16 to detect an additional patient with dysplasia if using CE with targeted biopsy. Compared with white light, the use of CE added almost 11 minutes to the total procedure time, which also included the time spent on random biopsies.

Improvements in detection and visualization of dysplasia in patients with IBD have led to an increase in their local endoscopic resection, without the need for colectomy,[34] all emphasizing the importance of careful and complete surveillance colonoscopies in these high-risk patients. Although CE is increasingly recommended for this purpose,[35,36] it has yet to be widely adopted as standard of care in clinical practice. Some of the reasons for this may be because CE is perceived as time consuming and often messy. These and perhaps additional factors like differences in application technique (spray catheter vs foot pump), dye contact time, operator experience, and interpretation of staining are the important training ingredients to broadly implement CE into routine clinical practice. Picco and colleagues[31] have shown excellent interobserver agreement among nonexpert endoscopists in the detection and interpretation of lesions detected by CE and the suggested steps toward training a unit to implement CE.

High-Definition Electronic Image-Enhanced Endoscopy (Virtual Chromoendoscopy)

CE with indigo carmine or methylene blue has been well demonstrated and is now incorporated into surveillance guidelines.[21] However, the perceived increased effort, skill, time, and cost of CE have motivated studies on electronic-based image-enhanced endoscopy or dyeless virtual CE. Three different systems are commercially available: Narrow Band imaging (NBI, Olympus, Tokyo, Japan), Fujinon Intelligent Color Enhancement (FICE, Fujifilm, Tokyo, Japan), and i-scan (Pentax, Tokyo, Japan). The basic principle of all these enhancement techniques is to filter the classical white light images to enhance superficial structural and vascular changes in the mucosa. In case of NBI, an optical filter is placed in front of the excitation white light source to narrow the wavelength to 30-nm bandwidths in the blue (415 nm) and green (540 nm) regions of the spectrum. Superficial mucosal structures (pit patterns) and microvasculature are enhanced using a narrow band light because it has more shallow tissue penetration and is mostly absorbed by hemoglobin in the vessels.

In contrast to NBI, the FICE and i-scan techniques do not use a physical filter but a postprocessing spectrum analysis software to enhance the image features and characteristics. The video processor disintegrates the different red green blue components of the white light image. Each component is then independently converted along its tone curve, followed by resynthesis of the 3 components to reconstruct a new digital image.[37–41] In theory, the number of possible combinations is endless, but each system comes with readily available filters. For example, the FICE system has 10 available filters, which can be activated by a push of the button and can be changed on the numeric key path of the processor's keyboard. Pentax has 3 major i-scan presets with standardized surface, tone, and contrast enhancement that come as a factory setting.

Because all these techniques are standardly available and can be simply activated by pushing a button, they have the appeal to overcome the technical drawbacks of

Table 2
Published studies comparing pancolonic chromoendoscopy with white light endoscopy in detection of dysplastic lesions for surveillance colonoscopy in long-standing colonic IBD

Author, Year	Country	No. of Endoscopists	Dye	Study Design	Inclusion Criteria	No. of Patients	No. with Dysplasia	Was CE Better[a]
Kiesslich et al,[11] 2003	Germany	Multiple	MB	Randomized 1:1	Long-standing UC ≥8 y	165	18	Y
Matsumoto et al,[12] 2003	Japan	Single	IC	Prospective cohort, WLE followed by CE	Pancolitis >5 y	57	12	Y
Rutter et al,[13] 2004	UK	Single	IC	Prospective cohort, WLE followed by CE	Long-standing extensive UC	100	7	Y
Kiesslich et al,[14] 2007	Germany	Multiple	MB	Randomized 1:1	Long-standing UC ≥8 y	153	15	Y
Marion et al,[17] 2008	USA	Multiple	MB	Prospective cohort, WLE followed by CE	Extensive UC or Crohn's colitis involving >1/3 of colon	102	22	Y
Günther et al,[29] 2011	Germany	Multiple	IC	Subdivided retrospectively into 50 patients in each group	Extensive UC >8 y or colonic Crohn's colitis >10 y	100	2	N
Hlavaty et al,[30] 2011	Slovakia	Multiple	IC	Retrospective analysis based on consent for WLE alone or WLE followed by CE	Pancolitis >8 y or left sided colitis >15 y	45	6	Y
Picco et al,[31] 2013	USA	Multiple	IC	Prospective cohort WLE followed by CE	Long standing extensive UC >8 y	75	16	Y

Abbreviations: IC, indigo carmine; MB, methylene blue; N, no; Y, yes.
[a] Detection by CE was significantly ($P<.05$) better than by WLE.

dye-based CE. In non-IBD settings, the diagnostic accuracy of NBI, FICE, and i-scan in discriminating neoplastic from nonneoplastic lesions is comparable to dye-based CE,[42–46] and at least this aspect of the technique seems to have a short learning curve.[47,48]

To date, the only electronic image-enhanced endoscopic technique to be assessed for diagnostic accuracy in IBD, however, has been using NBI. Five randomized trials[15,18,19,49,50] using NBI compared with CE ($n = 2$) or white light imaging ($n = 3$) did not show superiority in the detection of neoplastic lesions in long-standing colitis. Dekker and colleagues[15] showed no diagnostic advantage in a tandem colonoscopic study that compared the first-generation NBI system to standard-resolution WLE for the detection of colitis-associated neoplasia. NBI detected 52 visible lesions in 17 patients (8 neoplastic), compared with 28 visible lesions in 13 patients (7 neoplastic) during WLE inspection. Two more trials comparing HD-NBI to WLE also found no significant difference in the detection of neoplastic lesions when using NBI. Van den Broek and colleagues[18] performed a tandem colonoscopy study and found 13 of 16 (81%) neoplastic lesions using HD-NBI compared with 11 of 16 (69%) neoplastic lesions using HD-WLE.[18] Random biopsy protocol yielded no significant additional neoplasia; in a total of 1590 random biopsies, 3 demonstrated low-grade dysplasia of which 2 were found in the proximity of dysplasia associated lesion or mass lesions. Ignjatovic and colleagues[19] assessed the diagnostic yield of HD-NBI compared with WLE in a randomized controlled trial without back-to-back design and could not find a significant difference in neoplasia detection between the 2 techniques (5 neoplastic lesions in 5 patients for HD-NBI vs 7 neoplastic lesions in 5 patients for HD-WLE). Only 1 in 2707 random biopsies yielded an additional diagnosis of low-grade dysplasia in a patient who already had a lesion detected by NBI-targeted biopsies.[19] These studies add further to the evidence random biopsies are low yield and should be abandoned.[18,19,51]

Two trials have compared HD-NBI to CE. In a back-to-back study,[49] 33 patients underwent HD colonoscopy with NBI followed by CE (0.5% indigo carmine) and 27 patients were randomized to the opposite sequence to assess miss rates of the 2 techniques. The study showed a nonsignificant trend toward a higher miss rate using NBI. In the NBI first group, NBI detected 7 neoplastic lesions in 4 patients during the first pass and CE detected 5 additional lesions in 4 patients during the second pass. In the HD-CE first group, CE detected 5 neoplastic lesions in 4 patients during the first pass and NBI detected 3 neoplastic lesions in 1 patient during the second pass. The withdrawal time for CE was significantly longer (26.87 ± 9.89 minutes for CE vs 15.74 ± 5.62 minutes for NBI, $P<.01$).[49] Preliminary abstract data of a randomized trial comparing HD-NBI with CE (0.1% methylene blue) showed no significant difference in neoplasia detection rates between either modalities (18.5% for HD-NBI and 16.7% for HD-CE, $P = .658$).[50]

At present, CE remains the gold standard for colitis surveillance. Further studies assessing NBI or other electronic image-enhanced endoscopic methods compared with CE are necessary before any change in recommendations or clinical practice.

Autofluorescence Imaging

Autofluorescence imaging (AFI) is a novel imaging technique. AFI is available on the monochrome chip (Lucera, Olympus, Tokyo, Japan), which has 2 charge-coupled devices for WLE and AFI and can be activated by a push of the button. An ultraviolet filter is placed in front of the light source. All tissues exhibit autofluorescence when excited by ultraviolet (>400 nm) or short visible light (400–550 nm). Autofluorescence is generated by fluorophores, certain biomolecules (collagen, elastin), emitting a longer wavelength than the excitation light. AFI is influenced by several factors, including tissue architecture (mucosal thickening), light absorption and scattering properties (mainly determined by the absorptive capacity of hemoglobin in neoplastic neovascularization), the biochemical content (concentration of fluorophores), and metabolic status of the tissue.[52–59] Using AFI, neoplastic tissue is visible as a purple lesion on a greenish background fluorescence of normal colonic tissue. AFI has therefore the potential to serve as a red flag technique highlighting even very early minute neoplastic changes in the colonic mucosa. In contrast to NBI, the available data on AFI for colitis surveillance is sparse. In a single prospective randomized crossover trial comparing the neoplasia detection of WLE with that of AFI targeted biopsies, Van den Broek and colleagues[16] found a significant higher yield for AFI. In the AFI first group, 10 lesions in 25 patients were detected and subsequent WLE did not detect any additional lesions. However, in the WLE first group, 3 neoplastic lesions were detected in 25 patients, but AFI additionally detected 3 lesions. This resulted in a significantly different miss rate (50% vs 0, $P = .036$) between the 2 techniques.[16] Further larger trials are needed to confirm the potential of this red flag technique and to compare its yield with that of CE-guided biopsies.

SUMMARY

Patients with long-standing extensive colitis are at increased risk for developing neoplasia and the literature suggests that surveillance endoscopy reduces mortality from CRC in these patients. CE with indigo carmine or methylene blue has replaced random biopsies as a standard for surveillance in these patients; this is supported by several clinical trials and incorporated in recent guidelines. Future studies on digitally enhanced imaging, such as NBI, will continue to be of interest, but one has to be cautious that current data do not show their superiority compared with CE.

Future unmet needs in colitis surveillance include proper training and implementation for all endoscopists. Although the evidence is abundant and supports the use of CE, it is far from being widely implemented outside of tertiary referral centers. The minimal criteria need to be standardized to determine properly trained endoscopists. An endoscopist may need to start with CE coupled with 4-quadrant biopsies and then cautiously proceed with CE-guided biopsies once competence metrics are met. The implementation of these techniques needs to be monitored in prospective quality registries to ensure patient safety and the performance by secondary care gastroenterologists.

REFERENCES

1. Eaden JA, Abrams KR, Mayberry JF. The risk of colorectal cancer in ulcerative colitis: a meta-analysis. Gut 2001;48:526–35.
2. Carter MJ, Lobo AJ, Travis SP. Guidelines for the management of inflammatory bowel disease in adults. Gut 2004;53(Suppl 5):V1–16.
3. Kornbluth A, Sachar DB. Ulcerative colitis practice guidelines in adults (update): American College of Gastroenterology, Practice Parameters Committee. Am J Gastroenterol 2004;99:1371–85.
4. Rutter MD, Saunders BP, Wilkinson KH, et al. Thirty-year analysis of a colonoscopic surveillance program for neoplasia in ulcerative colitis. Gastroenterology 2006;130:1030–8.
5. Delaunoit T, Limburg PJ, Goldberg RM, et al. Colorectal cancer prognosis among patients with inflammatory bowel disease. Clin Gastroenterol Hepatol 2006;4:335–42.

6. Lakatos L, Mester G, Erdelyi Z, et al. Risk factors for ulcerative colitis-associated colorectal cancer in a Hungarian cohort of patients with ulcerative colitis: results of a population-based study. Inflamm Bowel Dis 2006;12:205–11.

7. Choi PM, Nugent FW, Schoetz DJ Jr, et al. Colonoscopic surveillance reduces mortality from colorectal cancer in ulcerative colitis. Gastroenterology 1993; 105:418–24.

8. Collins PD, Mpofu C, Watson AJ, et al. Strategies for detecting colon cancer and/or dysplasia in patients with inflammatory bowel disease. Cochrane Database Syst Rev 2006;(2):CD000279.

9. Eaden JA, Ward BA, Mayberry JF. How gastroenterologists screen for colonic cancer in ulcerative colitis: an analysis of performance. Gastrointest Endosc 2000;51:123–8.

10. Rubin CE, Haggitt RC, Burmer GC, et al. DNA aneuploidy in colonic biopsies predicts future development of dysplasia in ulcerative colitis. Gastroenterology 1992;103:1611–20.

11. Kiesslich R, Fritsch J, Holtmann M, et al. Methylene blue-aided chromoendoscopy for the detection of intraepithelial neoplasia and colon cancer in ulcerative colitis. Gastroenterology 2003;124:880–8.

12. Matsumoto T, Nakamura S, Jo Y, et al. Chromoscopy might improve diagnostic accuracy in cancer surveillance for ulcerative colitis. Am J Gastroenterol 2003; 98:1827–33.

13. Rutter MD, Saunders BP, Schofield G, et al. Pancolonic indigo carmine dye spraying for the detection of dysplasia in ulcerative colitis. Gut 2004;53:256–60.

14. Kiesslich R, Goetz M, Lammersdorf K, et al. Chromoscopy-guided endomicroscopy increases the diagnostic yield of intraepithelial neoplasia in ulcerative colitis. Gastroenterology 2007;132:874–82.

15. Dekker E, van den Broek FJ, Reitsma JB, et al. Narrow-band imaging compared with conventional colonoscopy for the detection of dysplasia in patients with longstanding ulcerative colitis. Endoscopy 2007;39:216–21.

16. van den Broek FJC, Fockens P, van Eeden S, et al. Endoscopic tri-modal imaging for surveillance in ulcerative colitis: randomised comparison of high-resolution endoscopy and autofluorescence imaging for neoplasia detection; and evaluation of narrow-band imaging for classification of lesions. Gut 2008; 57:1083–9.

17. Marion JF, Waye JD, Present DH, et al. Chromoendoscopy-targeted biopsies are superior to standard colonoscopic surveillance for detecting dysplasia in inflammatory bowel disease patients: a prospective endoscopic trial. Am J Gastroenterol 2008;103:2342–9.

18. van den Broek FJC, Fockens P, van Eeden S, et al. Narrow-band imaging versus high-definition endoscopy for the diagnosis of neoplasia in ulcerative colitis. Endoscopy 2011;43:108–15.

19. Ignjatovic A, East JE, Subramanian V, et al. Narrow band imaging for detection of dysplasia in colitis: a randomized controlled trial. Am J Gastroenterol 2012; 107:885–90.

20. van den Broek FJ, Stokkers PC, Reitsma JB, et al. Random biopsies taken during colonoscopic surveillance of patients with longstanding ulcerative colitis: low yield and absence of clinical consequences. Am J Gastroenterol 2011. [Epub ahead of print].

21. Cairns SR, Scholefield JH, Steele RJ, et al. Guidelines for colorectal cancer screening and surveillance in moderate and high risk groups (update from 2002). Gut 2010;59:666–89.

22. Annese V, Daperno M, Rutter MD, et al. European evidence based consensus for endoscopy in inflammatory bowel disease. J Crohns Colitis 2013;7: 982–1018.
23. Olliver JR, Wild CP, Sahay P, et al. Chromoendoscopy with methylene blue and associated DNA damage in Barrett's oesophagus. Lancet 2003;362:373–4.
24. Davies J, Burke D, Olliver JR, et al. Methylene blue but not indigo carmine causes DNA damage to colonocytes in vitro and in vivo at concentrations used in clinical chromoendoscopy. Gut 2007;56:155–6.
25. Huneburg R, Lammert F, Rabe C, et al. Chromocolonoscopy detects more adenomas than white light colonoscopy or narrow band imaging colonoscopy in hereditary nonpolyposis colorectal cancer screening. Endoscopy 2009;41: 316–22.
26. Le Rhun M, Coron E, Parlier D, et al. High resolution colonoscopy with chromoscopy versus standard colonoscopy for the detection of colonic neoplasia: a randomized study. Clin Gastroenterol Hepatol 2006;4:349–54.
27. Rubin DT, Rothe JA, Hetzel JT, et al. Are dysplasia and colorectal cancer endoscopically visible in patients with ulcerative colitis? Gastrointest Endosc 2007; 65:998–1004.
28. Rutter MD, Saunders BP, Wilkinson KH, et al. Most dysplasia in ulcerative colitis is visible at colonoscopy. Gastrointest Endosc 2004;60:334–9.
29. Günther U, Kusch D, Heller F, et al. Surveillance colonoscopy in patients with inflammatory bowel disease: comparison of random biopsy vs. targeted biopsy protocols. Int J Colorectal Dis 2011;26:667–72.
30. Hlavaty T, Huorka M, Koller T, et al. Colorectal cancer screening in patients with ulcerative and Crohn's colitis with use of colonoscopy, chromoendoscopy and confocal endomicroscopy. Eur J Gastroenterol Hepatol 2011;23: 680–9.
31. Picco MF, Pasha S, Leighton JA, et al. Procedure time and the determination of polypoid abnormalities with experience: implementation of a chromoendoscopy program for surveillance colonoscopy for ulcerative colitis. Inflamm Bowel Dis 2013;19:1913–20.
32. Subramanian V, Mannath J, Ragunath K, et al. Meta-analysis: the diagnostic yield of chromoendoscopy for detecting dysplasia in patients with colonic inflammatory bowel disease. Aliment Pharmacol Ther 2011;33:304–12.
33. Soetikno R, Subramanian V, Kaltenbach T, et al. The detection of nonpolypoid (flat and depressed) colorectal neoplasms in patients with inflammatory bowel disease. Gastroenterology 2013;144:1349–52, 1352.
34. Hurlstone DP, Sanders DS, Atkinson R, et al. Endoscopic mucosal resection for flat neoplasia in chronic ulcerative colitis: can we change the endoscopic management paradigm? Gut 2007;56:838–46.
35. Itzkowitz SH, Harpaz N. Diagnosis and management of dysplasia in patients with inflammatory bowel diseases. Gastroenterology 2004;126:1634–48.
36. Hayashi N, Tanaka S, Hewett DG, et al. Endoscopic prediction of deep submucosal invasive carcinoma: validation of the narrow-band imaging international colorectal endoscopic (NICE) classification. Gastrointest Endosc 2013;78: 625–32.
37. Kodashima S, Fujishiro M. Novel image-enhanced endoscopy with i-scan technology. World J Gastroenterol 2010;16:1043–9.
38. Adler A, Aschenbeck J, Yenerim T, et al. Narrow-band versus white-light high definition television endoscopic imaging for screening colonoscopy: a prospective randomized trial. Gastroenterology 2009;136:410–6.

39. Hoffman A, Sar F, Goetz M, et al. High definition colonoscopy combined with i-Scan is superior in the detection of colorectal neoplasias compared with standard video colonoscopy: a prospective randomized controlled trial. Endoscopy 2010;42(10):827–33.

40. Hoffman A, Kagel C, Goetz M, et al. Recognition and characterization of small colonic neoplasia with high-definition colonoscopy using i-Scan is as precise as chromoendoscopy. Dig Liver Dis 2010;42(1):45–50.

41. Rex DK, Helbig CC. High yields of small and flat adenomas with high-definition colonoscopes using either white light or narrow band imaging. Gastroenterology 2007;133(1):42–7.

42. Hewett DG, Kaltenbach T, Sano Y, et al. Validation of a simple classification system for endoscopic diagnosis of small colorectal polyps using narrow-band imaging. Gastroenterology 2012;143:599–607.

43. Basford PJ, Longcroft-Wheaton G, Higgins B, et al. High-definition endoscopy with i-Scan for evaluation of small colon polyps: the HiSCOPE study. Gastrointest Endosc 2014;79:111–8.

44. Longcroft-Wheaton G, Brown J, Cowlishaw D, et al. High-definition vs standard-definition colonoscopy in the characterization of small colonic polyps: results from a randomized trial. Endoscopy 2012;44:905–10.

45. Longcroft-Wheaton GR, Higgins B, Bhandari P. Flexible spectral imaging color enhancement and indigo carmine in neoplasia diagnosis during colonoscopy: a large prospective UK series. Eur J Gastroenterol Hepatol 2011;23:903–11.

46. Pohl J, Nguyen-Tat M, Pech O, et al. Computed virtual chromoendoscopy for classification of small colorectal lesions: a prospective comparative study. Am J Gastroenterol 2008;103:562–9.

47. Bouwens MW, de RR, Masclee AA, et al. Optical diagnosis of colorectal polyps using high-definition i-scan: an educational experience. World J Gastroenterol 2013;19:4334–43.

48. Neumann H, Vieth M, Fry LC, et al. Learning curve of virtual chromoendoscopy for the prediction of hyperplastic and adenomatous colorectal lesions: a prospective 2-center study. Gastrointest Endosc 2013;78(1):115–20.

49. Pellisé M, López-Cerón M, Rodríguez de Miguel C, et al. Narrow-band imaging as an alternative to chromoendoscopy for the detection of dysplasia in long-standing inflammatory bowel disease: a prospective, randomized, crossover study. Gastrointest Endosc 2011;74:840–8.

50. Bisschops R, Bessissow T, Baert FJ, et al. Chromo-endoscopy versus narrow band imaging in ulcerative colitis: a prospective randomized controlled trial. Gastrointest Endosc 2012;44:AB148.

51. Subramanian V, Ramappa V, Telakis E, et al. Comparison of high definition with standard white light endoscopy for detection of dysplastic lesions during surveillance colonoscopy in patients with inflammatory bowel disease. Inflamm Bowel Dis 2013;19:350–5.

52. DaCosta RS, Andersson H, Wilson BC. Molecular fluorescence excitation-emission matrices relevant to tissue spectroscopy. Photochem Photobiol 2003;78:384–92.

53. DaCosta RS, Wilson BC, Marcon NE. Optical techniques for the endoscopic detection of dysplastic colonic lesions. Curr Opin Gastroenterol 2005;21(1):70–9.

54. Matsumoto T, Nakamura S, Moriyama T, et al. Autofluorescence imaging colonoscopy for the detection of dysplastic lesions in ulcerative colitis: a pilot study. Colorectal Dis 2010;12:e291–7.

55. Bessissow T, Bisschops R. Advanced endoscopic imaging for dysplasia surveillance in ulcerative colitis. Expert Rev Gastroenterol Hepatol 2013;7:57–67.
56. Neumann H, Neurath MF, Mudter J. New endoscopic approaches in IBD. World J Gastroenterol 2011;17(1):63–8.
57. Subramanian V, Ragunath K. Advanced endoscopic imaging: a review of commercially available technologies. Clin Gastroenterol Hepatol 2014;12: 368–76.e1 pii:S1542–3565(13)00878-1.
58. van den Broek FJ, van Es JA, van Eeden S, et al. Pilot study of probe-based confocal laser endomicroscopy during colonoscopic surveillance of patients with longstanding ulcerative colitis. Endoscopy 2011;43:116–22.
59. Jess T, Loftus EV Jr, Velayos FS, et al. Incidence and prognosis of colorectal dysplasia in inflammatory bowel disease: a population-based study from Olmsted County, Minnesota. Inflamm Bowel Dis 2006;12(8):669–76.

Detection of Nonpolypoid Colorectal Neoplasia Using Magnifying Endoscopy in Colonic Inflammatory Bowel Disease

(®) CrossMark

Shiro Oka, MD, PhD[a], Shinji Tanaka, MD, PhD[a],*,
Kazuaki Chayama, MD, PhD[b]

KEYWORDS

- Colitis-associated dysplasia/cancer • Inflammatory bowel disease
- Ulcerative colitis • Image-enhanced endoscopy • Narrow band imaging
- Autofluorescence imaging • Magnifying endoscopy

KEY POINTS

- Most nonpolypoid colorectal neoplasms (NP-CRNs) are visible, and their detection can be facilitated by the use of chromoendoscopy.
- Chromoendoscopy using indigo carmine, in turn, also augments our further evaluation of the border and pit pattern of the lesion.
- Magnifying endoscopy can assist us to further visualize the surface pattern, although chronic inflammation and its sequela in patients with inflammatory bowel disease (IBD) make the use of the pit pattern analysis less useful.
- In Japan, at present, efforts are given to clarify the merit for random biopsy.
- A nationwide randomized controlled trial is ongoing to clarify whether target biopsy or random step biopsy is effective for the detection of NP-CRN.

INTRODUCTION

Patients with inflammatory bowel disease (IBD) have a high risk of colitis-associated dysplasia and cancer.[1,2] These types of dysplasia and cancer, as compared with sporadic adenoma/carcinoma, seem to have a distinct growth pattern, which can be flat,

Disclosure of interests: None of the authors have any financial relationships to disclose relevant to this publication.
[a] Department of Endoscopy, Hiroshima University Hospital, 1-2-3 Kasumi, Minami-ku, Hiroshima 734-8551, Japan; [b] Department of Gastroenterology and Metabolism, Hiroshima University, Hospital, 1-2-3 Kasumi, Minami-ku, Hiroshima 734-8551, Japan
* Corresponding author.
E-mail address: colon@hiroshima-u.ac.jp

multifocal, or anaplastic.[3–7] Therefore, it is important that careful surveillance with co-lonoscopy is performed for all patients with IBD and, more frequently, for those considered to be at high risk.[8–12] Traditionally, flat dysplasia in ulcerative colitis (UC) has been considered to be detectable only by using random biopsy specimens of mucosa that appeared unremarkable during endoscopy.[13–15] However, recent studies have shown that most of them are visible; thus, their detection as nonpolypoid colorectal neoplasms (NP-CRNs) is an integral component in the prevention of colitic cancer.[9,16–18]

Unlike dysplasia-associated lesions or masses, which are readily visible using conventional endoscopy,[19] the detection of NP-CRN can be more difficult. NP-CRN in colitic IBD (cIBD) is often present simply as redness or a granular patch of mucosa that may not be readily distinguishable from the surrounding inflamed mucosa. Because it is often difficult to identify NP-CRN in cIBD using white light endoscopy, random blind biopsies are still commonly practiced, especially in Western countries, to potentially help detect these lesions. An alternative to random biopsy is to enhance the appearance of NP-CRN by using image-enhanced endoscopy and, in turn, to target the biopsy on areas that appear abnormal.

Several recent trials have evaluated dye-based image enhanced endoscopy (chromoendoscopy),[20–28] magnifying endoscopy,[16,29–33] and equipment-based image-enhanced endoscopy (IEE)[34–45] to detect NP-CRN in cIBD. Of these techniques, the indigo carmine dye spray IEE has been shown to effectively increase the detection of areas suspected to contain NP-CRN and to delineate the border and surface of suspected and obvious lesions.[46] Equipment-based IEE is a promising, but unproven, method that is designed to visualize small vessels and minute mucosal patterns. Of the currently available equipment-based IEE: narrow band imaging [NBI; Olympus, Tokyo, Japan], flexible spectral imaging color enhancement [Fujifilm, Tokyo, Japan], blue laser image [Fujifilm, Tokyo, Japan], autofluorescence imaging [AFI; Olympus, Tokyo, Japan], and i-scan [Pentax, Tokyo, Japan], clinical trials on the diagnosis of NP-CRN in cIBD have been published only for NBI and AFI.[34–45]

In this article, the authors describe the present status of the use of IEE to diagnose NP-CRN using magnifying colonoscope and illustrate their practice at the Hiroshima University Hospital. The authors have collated a few cases to provide examples of their practice. The authors do not reiterate data reporting on the utility of chromoendoscopy as Subramanian and Bisschops have summarized them.

THE PREVALENCE OF NP-CRN IN PATIENTS WITH IBD

Data show that nonpolypoid colorectal lesions are common in patients with IBD. The true prevalence of NP-CRN in UC is difficult to estimate with the present endoscopic modality. Several studies provide a general estimate. Sada and colleagues[16] reported that with surveillance colonoscopy in 1115 patients with UC, 39 colitic dysplasias or cancers in 31 patients were detected; 30% of dysplasias (6 of 20) were flat, and 16% of cancers (3 of 19) were depressed lesions. Toruner and colleagues[17] reported that among 635 patients with IBD, 36 dysplasias were detected; 24 (67%) were nonpolypoid and 12 (33%) were polypoid. Rutter and colleagues[18] reported that 77% of 110 colitic dysplasias or cancers in 525 patients with UC were detected endoscopically, with 23% being flat. In an investigation by the Japanese Ministry of Health, Labor, and Welfare, 42 lesions (79%) were polypoid and 11 lesions (21%) were nonpolypoid. Other reports have shown that more NP-CRN were detected and diagnosed using magnifying endoscopy as compared with chromoendoscopy.[16,28–33]

DETECTION OF NP-CRN WITH CHROMOENDOSCOPY

The recent use of high-definition endoscopy with chromoendoscopy has enabled endoscopists to directly visualize, localize, and diagnose NP-CRN in patients with UC (see **Table 1**). Indigo carmine solution enhances the visualization of the border and surface topography of the lesion to improve contrast compared with the surrounding mucosa in patients with UC.[46] A meta-analysis has demonstrated that chromoendoscopy has medium to high sensitivity (83.3%, 95% confidence interval [CI]: 35.9–99.6), specificity (91.3%, 95% CI: 43.8–100), and high diagnostic accuracy (odds ratio 17.544, 95% CI: 1.245–247.14) for dysplastic lesions[47] and is superior to white light colonoscopy for the proportion of lesions detected by biopsies (44%, 95% CI: 28.6–59.1) as well as for flat dysplasia (27%, 95% CI: 11.2–41.9) in patients with UC.[26]

Kiesslich and colleagues[20] reported 165 patients with long-standing UC who were randomized to conventional colonoscopy or colonoscopy with chromoendoscopy using 0.1% methylene blue. More targeted biopsies were possible, and significant intraepithelial neoplasia was detected in the chromoendoscopy group (32 vs 10; $P = .003$). Rutter and colleagues[23] reported the importance of indigo carmine dye spraying for the detection of dysplasia in UC. They emphasized that no dysplasia was detected in 2904 nontargeted biopsies. In comparison, chromoendoscopy with targeted biopsy led to fewer biopsies and detected 9 dysplastic lesions, 7 of which were only visible after indigo carmine application. They concluded that the indigo carmine dye spraying of the whole colon is feasible, and dysplasia detection may be more effective than taking large numbers of random biopsies. Hurlstone and colleagues[31] also emphasized that indigo carmine–assisted high-magnification chromoendoscopy and improved the detection of intraepithelial neoplasia in the endoscopic screening of patients with UC.

However, pancolonic chromoendoscopy has potential limitations: dye on the mucosa is not always equally spread; dye pooling can lead to difficult observation; more time is needed; and some biopsies may be false negative.

In the authors' institution, they routinely perform high-magnification colonoscopy with indigo carmine chromoendoscopy after they suspect the presence of NP-CRN in patients with cIBD. Morphologically, NP-CRN in IBD appear to be slightly elevated, completely flat, or slightly depressed as compared with the surrounding mucosa. In order to detect them, the authors look for the presence of a slightly elevated lesion, focal friability, obscure vascular pattern, discoloration (uneven redness or a patch or redness), villous mucosa (velvety appearance), and irregular nodularity. The finding of any of these signs typically alerts the authors to become suspicious of the possible presence of NP-CRN and leads them to wash out the mucus or debris from the surface on the target lesion and apply the dye for magnifying colonoscopy.[15]

MAGNIFYING COLONOSCOPY USING DYE SPRAYING FOR NP-CRN

After dye spraying but before the authors perform a biopsy or resection, they will typically evaluate the border of the lesion. The authors look for the presence of dye pooling within the lesion, which would suggest the diagnosis of a depressed lesions. The authors study the pit pattern of the mucosal surface.[15] The authors' experience and others', however, suggest that the current pit pattern classification may not be completely applicable in UC, because the pit pattern of the regenerative hyperplastic villous mucosa in UC (with the pits becoming elongated and irregular, depending on the degree of inflammation) is difficult to distinguish from neoplastic pit patterns. Instead of using the current pit pattern classification,[48] the authors have previously reported that high residual density of pits and irregular pit margins with magnification

Table 1
Studies on the use of chromoendoscopy in IBD

Author, Published Year	No. of Patients	Study Design	Setting	Dye (%)	Endoscopy Compared	Indication	Main Outcomes	Statistics: P Value for Comparison
Kiesslich et al,[20] 2003	165	Parallel randomized trial	UC surveillance	MB 0.1	WLE	Dysplasia detection	True-positive lesions, CE 32 vs WLE 10	.00315
Matsumoto et al,[21] 2003	57	Prospective study	UC surveillance	IC 0.2	WLE	Dysplasia detection	Sensitivity, CE 86% vs WLE 38%	NS
Rutter et al,[23] 2004	100	Prospective study	UC surveillance	IC 0.1	WLE	Dysplasia detection	True-positive lesions, CE 9 vs WLE 2	.06
Hurlstone et al,[31] 2005	81	Prospective study	UC surveillance	IC 0.5	WLE	Dysplasia detection	True-positive lesions, CE 69 vs WLE 24	<.0001
Kiesslich et al,[9] 2007	153	Parallel randomized trial	UC surveillance	MB 0.1	WLE	Dysplasia detection	True-positive lesions, CE 19 vs WLE 4	.005
Marion et al,[25] 2008	102	Cross-sectional study	IBD surveillance	MB 0.1	WLE	Dysplasia detection	True-positive patients, CE 17 vs WLE 3	.001
Günther et al,[27] 2011	150	Parallel randomized trial	IBD surveillance	IC 0.1	WLE	Dysplasia detection	True-positive patients, CE 6 vs WLE 0	<.05

Abbreviations: CE, chromoendoscopy; IC, indigo carmine; MB, methylene blue; NS, not significant; WLE, white light endoscopy.

after indigo carmine dye spraying were useful to differentiate between colitis-associated neoplastic and non-neoplastic lesions.[33] Therefore, in the authors' practice, they focus on the high residual density of pits and irregular pit margins observed under magnifying chromocolonoscopy.[33]

The main pit patterns of neoplasia in cIBD have been reported as type IV and type III_S with a III_L pit pattern. Sada and colleagues[16] described that magnifying colonoscopy of 15 neoplasias and showed that the patterns being type III_S- to III_L or type IV pit. Hata and colleagues[30] reported that they found no neoplastic lesions in regions characterized by type II or I pit patterns. However, they also noted that some non-neoplastic flat lesions also have type III and IV pit patterns, which are neoplastic patterns. After completion of the characterization of the lesion, the authors perform the biopsy or remove the lesion.

DETECTION OF NP-CRN USING EQUIPMENT-BASED IEE
NBI

NBI is commonly used for the management of colorectal lesions in Japan. A large body of the literature has reported on the utility of NBI for the detection of colorectal polyps[49–54] and for differentiating the diagnosis between neoplastic and non-neoplastic lesions.[49,55–61] Conversely, some studies have suggested that NBI magnification is not effective for the detection of colorectal neoplasia.[62–66] An advantage of NBI magnification is that it can be achieved without spraying dye, thus potentially reducing the cost. Because NBI involves a simple one-touch operation, NBI magnification may shorten the procedure time required for diagnosing NP-CRN in IBD and make the surveillance colonoscopy efficient. The major limitation of NBI, however, is that the visual field becomes too dark during its application. A newer generation of NBI has, therefore, been developed with improved brightness, although prospective trials have not been performed.

In the previous clinical research on the significance of NBI endoscopy in detecting NP-CRN in patients with UC, surveillance colonoscopy using NBI was associated with negative results[34–37]; no significant difference in the ability to detect NP-CRN was found between NBI and white light endoscopy (**Table 2**). Dekker and colleagues[35] reported that 52 visible lesions were identified in 17 patients during NBI endoscopy compared with 28 visible lesions identified in patients using white light endoscopy. A pathologic evaluation of target biopsies showed 11 patients with neoplasia, which was detected by both techniques in 4 patients, whereas only 4 cases were detected using NBI endoscopy alone and 3 cases using white light endoscopy. Van den Broek and colleagues[38] also reported that 11 of 16 (69%) neoplastic lesions were detected by white light, whereas NBI endoscopy detected 13 of 16 (81%) cases (nonsignificant differences). Efthymiou and colleagues[42] reported that when using chromoendoscopy, 131 lesions (92%) were detected as compared with 102 lesions (70%) with NBI ($P<.001$); the median number of lesions detected per patient was 3 with chromoendoscopy and 1.5 with NBI ($P = .002$).

NBI magnification, however, was not used in these clinical studies. The authors, thus, have continued to study the use of magnifying endoscopy with NBI in their unit in Hiroshima (**Figs. 1–3**). The authors think that it is possible that the reported results in the literature were negative because of the difficulty to accurately discriminate between active inflammation and neoplasia. The authors also studied other potential advantages of the use of NBI magnification. Bisschops and colleagues[40] reported that the withdrawal time for NBI was significantly shorter than that of CE, although NBI endoscopy and CE showed equivalent dysplasia detection rates. Pellisé and

Table 2
Studies on the use of image-enhanced endoscopy in IBD

Author, Published Year	No. of Patients	Study Design	Setting	IEE	Endoscopy Compared	Indication	Main Outcomes	Statistics: P Value for Comparison
Dekker et al,[35] 2007	42	Randomized crossover trial	UC surveillance	NBI	WLE	Dysplasia detection	Suspicious lesions, NBI 52 vs WLE 28 True-positive lesions, NBI 9 vs WLE 12 False-positive lesions, NBI 43 vs WLE 16	.026 .672 .015
Matsumoto et al,[36] 2007	46	Cross-sectional study	UC surveillance	NBI	WLE	Dysplasia differentiation	Positive rate of dysplasia, tortuous pattern (4/50 sites, 8%) vs honeycomblike or villous patterns (1/246 sites, 0.4%)	.003
Van den Broek et al,[44] 2008	50	Randomized crossover trial	UC surveillance	AFI NBI	WLE AFI	Dysplasia detection Dysplasia differentiation	Neoplasia miss rates, AFI 0% vs and WLE 50% AFI (sensitivity 100%) vs NBI (sensitivity 75%, specificity 81%)	.036
Matsumoto et al,[43] 2010	48	Prospective study	UC surveillance	AFI	WLE	Dysplasia detection	Positive rate of dysplasia, protrusions (30%) vs flat mucosa (3.3%) Positive rate of dysplasia in flat lesions, low AF (8.2%) vs high AFI (0%)	<.0001 .3
Pellise et al,[37] 2011	60	Randomized crossover trial	UC surveillance	NBI	WLE with indigo carmine	Dysplasia detection	Suspicious lesions, NBI 136 vs WLE 208 True-positive lesions, NBI 10 vs WLE 12 False-positive lesions, NBI 126 vs WLI 196	.001 .644 .001
van den Broek et al,[38] 2011	48	Randomized crossover trial	IBD surveillance	NBI	WLE	Dysplasia detection	True-positive lesions, NBI 13 vs WLE 11	.727
Ignjatovic et al,[41] 2012	112	Parallel randomized trial	UC surveillance	NBI	WLE	Dysplasia detection	True-positive lesions, NBI 5 vs WLE 7 False-positive lesions, NBI 12 vs WLI 4	.57 .06
Efthymiou et al,[42] 2013	144	Randomized crossover trial	UC surveillance	NBI	WLE	Dysplasia detection	Suspicious lesions, NBI 102 vs WLE 131 True-positive lesions, NBI 20 vs WLE 23	<.001 .18

Abbreviation: WLE, white light endoscopy.

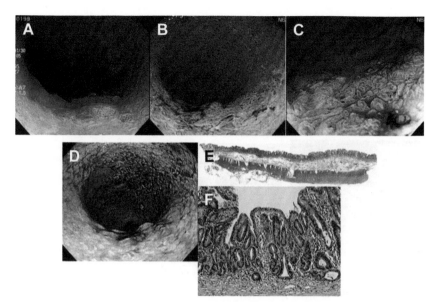

Fig. 1. A 53-year-old woman, 10 years after the onset of UC. (*A*) Ordinary colonoscopic view. A flat elevated lesion was noted in the rectum. (*B*) NBI showed the slightly elevated lesion with mucus present. (*C*) High-magnification imaging with NBI revealed the irregular surface pattern. (*D*) View with indigo carmine dye spraying. The focal lesion that is not covered with the indigo carmine solution is unclear. Proctocolectomy was performed. (*E*) Cross section of the specimen (hematoxylin-eosin). (*F*) The lesion was diagnosed histologically as intramucosal well-differentiated adenocarcinoma.

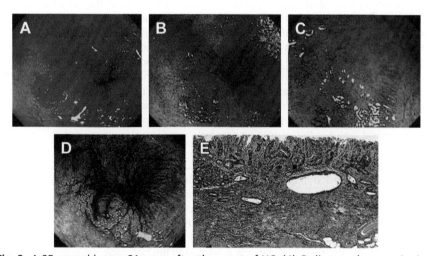

Fig. 2. A 35-year-old man, 21 years after the onset of UC. (*A*) Ordinary colonoscopic view. The reddened flat lesion was identified. (*B*) NBI showed the flat lesion as a brownish area. (*C*) High-magnification imaging with NBI revealed the irregular surface pattern and microvessels. (*D*) View with indigo carmine dye spraying. A 0-IIa+IIc lesion was clearly delineated. Proctocolectomy was performed. (*E*) The lesion was diagnosed histologically as submucosal invasive well-differentiated adenocarcinoma.

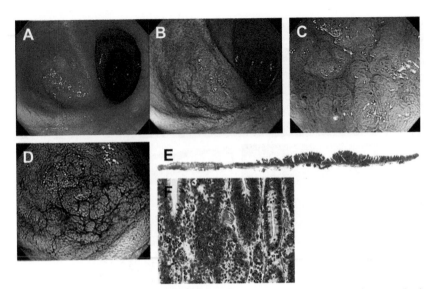

Fig. 3. A 47-year-old woman, 5 years after the onset of UC. (*A*) Ordinary colonoscopic view. A whitish flat elevated lesion was noted in the rectum. (*B*) NBI showed the slightly elevated lesion. (*C*) High-magnification imaging with NBI revealed the mild irregular surface pattern. (*D*) View with indigo carmine dye spraying. The focal lesion was relatively clear. Endoscopic submucosal dissection was performed on the lesion. (*E*) Cross section of the specimen (hematoxylin-eosin). (*F*) The lesion was diagnosed histologically as low-grade dysplasia.

colleagues[37] reported that NBI endoscopy had a significantly inferior false-positive biopsy rate and a similar true-positive rate compared with CE. It has been reported that the magnified observation of UC using NBI is useful to discriminate between dysplastic/neoplastic and non-neoplastic lesions and to guide for the necessity of performing a target biopsy. East and colleagues found that dysplasias were seen as darker capillary vascular patterns. Matsumoto and colleagues[36] reported that the tortuous pattern of capillaries determined by NBI endoscopy might be a clue for the identification of dysplasia during surveillance colonoscopy for patients with UC. The authors have previously reported the clinical usefulness of NBI magnification for the qualitative diagnosis of sporadic colorectal lesions by the combined evaluation of both surface pattern and microvessel features.[55] The surface pattern is thought to be more useful for endoscopic findings because inflammation causes the structure of microvessel features to become disordered.

AFI

AFI is a novel technique that uses a short-wavelength light to excite endogenous tissue fluorophores that emit fluorescent light of longer wavelength. AFI highlights neoplastic tissue without the administration of exogenous fluorophores as described earlier in UC.[43–45] AFI images of UC lesions can be classified into 4 categories: green, green with purple spots, purple with green spots, and purple. The strength of the purple staining in AFI images of UC lesions is related to the histologic severity. Using AFI, colitis-associated neoplasias are observed as a purple area, regardless of their macroscopic types.[43–45]

AFI endoscopy has been reported to be promising for the detection of dysplasia in UC,[43–45] although the clinical potential of AFI in routine colonoscopy has been complicated by high false-positive detection rates, particularly in cases of NP-CRN (see

Table 2). Van den Broek and colleagues[44] reported that AFI endoscopy improves the diagnosis of dysplasia in patients with UC. However, the interpretation of the results should be done with caution because the study initially excluded patients with active inflammation. Because AFI is attenuated in colonic inflammation as well as in neoplasm, such exclusion seems to have contributed positively to the assessment of AFI endoscopy by decreasing the number of false-positive areas. Matsumoto and colleagues[45] reported that AFI endoscopy identified 14 dysplasias in 4 patients during surveillance colonoscopy of 48 patients with UC. Eleven lesions were polypoid lesions, and the other 3 lesions were flat lesions. Autofluorescence as determined by AFI was regarded to be low in 12 lesions and to be normal in 2 lesions. Thus, the specificity of AFI endoscopy for the detection of flat dysplasia was, in fact, less than those of the prior investigations by NBI endoscopy or chromoendoscopy.[44,45] This finding seems to be a consequence of patchy inflammation in the observed area because autofluorescence under AFI endoscopy was altered according to the grade of inflammation in patients with UC. In order to use AFI for surveillance colonoscopy in patients with UC, it is necessary to express autofluorescence numerically and objectively and to clarify the discrimination between the inflammation and neoplastic lesions. There have not been any large trials on the usefulness of AFI for the detection of colitis-associated dysplasia and cancer. AFI may have great potential for the detection of non–polypoid colitis–associated dysplasia and cancer without magnification.

SUMMARY

Most NP-CRNs are visible, and their detection can be facilitated by the use of chromoendoscopy. Chromoendoscopy using indigo carmine, in turn, also augments the further evaluation of the border and surface pattern of the lesion. Magnifying endoscopy can assist in further visualizing the surface pattern, although chronic inflammation and its sequela in patients with IBD make the use of the pit pattern analysis less useful. In Japan, at present, efforts are given to clarify the merit for random biopsy. A nationwide randomized controlled trial is ongoing to clarify whether target biopsy or random step biopsy is effective for the detection of NP-CRN.[67]

REFERENCES

1. Collins PD, Mpofu C, Watson AJ, et al. Strategies for detecting colon cancer and/or dysplasia in patients with inflammatory bowel disease. Cochrane Database Syst Rev 2006;(2):CD000279.
2. Eaden JA, Abrams KR, Mayberry JF, et al. The risk of colorectal cancer in ulcerative colitis: a meta-analysis. Gut 2001;48:526–35.
3. Bernstein CN. Ulcerative colitis with low-grade dysplasia. Gastroenterology 2004;127:950–6.
4. Rutter MD, Saunders BP, Wilkinson KH, et al. Thirty-year analysis of a colonoscopic surveillance program for neoplasia in ulcerative colitis. Gastroenterology 2006;130:1030–8.
5. Hurlstone DP. The detection of flat and depressed colorectal lesions: which endoscopic imaging approach? Gastroenterology 2008;135:338–43.
6. Rutter M, Bernstein C, Matsumoto T, et al. Endoscopic appearance of dysplasia in ulcerative colitis and the role of staining. Endoscopy 2004;36:1109–14.
7. Farraye FA, Odze RD, Eaden J, et al. AGA technical review on the diagnosis and management of colorectal neoplasia in inflammatory bowel disease. Gastroenterology 2010;138:746–74.

8. Robertson DJ, Greenberg ER, Baron JA, et al. Colorectal cancer in patients under close colonoscopic surveillance. Gastroenterology 2005;129:34–41.

9. Kiesslich R, Goetz M, Lammersdorf K, et al. Chromoscopy-guided endomicroscopy increases the diagnostic yield of intraepithelial neoplasia in ulcerative colitis. Gastroenterology 2007;132:874–82.

10. Rex DK, Johnson DA, Anderson JC, et al. American College of Gastroenterology guidelines for colorectal cancer screening. Am J Gastroenterol 2009;104: 739–50.

11. Cairns SR, Scholefield JH, Steele RJ, et al. Guidelines for colorectal cancer screening and surveillance in moderate and high risk groups. Gut 2010;59:666–89.

12. Leung K, Pinsky P, Laiyemo AO, et al. Ongoing colorectal cancer risk despite surveillance colonoscopy: the Polyp Prevention Trial Continued Follow-up Study. Gastrointest Endosc 2010;71:111–7.

13. Tytgat GN, Dhir V, Gopinath N. Endoscopic appearance of dysplasia and cancer in inflammatory bowel disease. Eur J Cancer 1995;31A:1174–7.

14. Sharan R, Scoen RE. Cancer in inflammatory bowel disease. An evidence-based analysis and guide for physicians and patients. Gastroenterol Clin North Am 2002;31:237–54.

15. Ueno Y, Tanaka S, Chayama K. Non-polypoid colorectal neoplasms in ulcerative colitis. Gastrointest Endosc Clin N Am 2010;20:525–42.

16. Sada M, Igarashi M, Yoshizawa S, et al. Dye spraying and magnifying endoscopy for dysplasia and cancer surveillance in ulcerative colitis. Dis Colon Rectum 2004;47:1816–23.

17. Toruner M, Harewood GC, Loftus EV Jr, et al. Endoscopic factors in the diagnosis of colorectal dysplasia in chronic inflammatory bowel disease. Inflamm Bowel Dis 2005;11:428–34.

18. Rutter MD, Saunders BP, Wilkinson KH, et al. Most dysplasia in ulcerative colitis is visible at colonoscopy. Gastrointest Endosc 2004;60:334–9.

19. Blackstone MU, Riddle RF, Rogers BH, et al. Dysplasia-associated lesion or mass (DALM) detected by colonoscopy in long-standing ulcerative colitis; an indication for colectomy. Gastroenterology 1981;80:366–74.

20. Kiesslich R, Fritch J, Holtmann M, et al. Methylene-blue aided chromoendoscopy for the detection of intraepithelial neoplasia and colon cancer in ulcerative colitis. Gastroenterology 2003;124:880–8.

21. Matsumoto T, Nakamura S, Jo Y, et al. Chromoscopy might improve diagnostic accuracy in cancer surveillance for ulcerative colitis. Am J Gastroenterol 2003; 98:1827–33.

22. Kiesslich R, Neurath MF. Chromoendoscopy: an evolving standard in surveillance for ulcerative colitis. Inflamm Bowel Dis 2004;10:695–6.

23. Rutter MD, Saunders BP, Schofield G, et al. Pancolonic indigo carmine dye spraying for the detection of dysplasia in ulcerative colitis. Gut 2004;53:256–60.

24. Ullman TA. Chromoendoscopy should be the standard method and more widely used for cancer surveillance colonoscopy in ulcerative colitis. Inflamm Bowel Dis 2007;13:1273–4.

25. Marion JF, Waye JD, Present DH, et al. Chromoendoscopy-targeted biopsies are superior to standard colonoscopic surveillance for detecting dysplasia in inflammatory bowel disease patients: a prospective endoscopic trial. Am J Gastroenterol 2008;103:2342–9.

26. Subramanian V, Mannath J, Ragunath K, et al. Meta-analysis: the diagnostic yield of chromoendoscopy for detecting dysplasia in patients with colonic inflammatory bowel disease. Aliment Pharmacol Ther 2011;33:304–12.

27. Günther U, Kusch D, Heller F, et al. Surveillance colonoscopy in patients with inflammatory bowel disease: comparison of random biopsy vs. targeted biopsy protocols. Int J Colorectal Dis 2011;26:667–72.
28. Kiesslich R, Neurath MF. Chromoendoscopy in inflammatory bowel disease. Gastroenterol Clin North Am 2012;41:291–302.
29. Hurlstone DP, McAlindon ME, Sanders DS, et al. Further validation of high-magnification chromoscopic colonoscopy for the detection of intraepithelial neoplasia and colon cancer in ulcerative colitis. Gastroenterology 2004;126:376–8.
30. Hata K, Watanabe T, Motoi T, et al. Pitfalls of pit pattern diagnosis in ulcerative colitis-associated dysplasia. Gastroenterology 2004;126:374–6.
31. Hurlstone DP, Sanders DS, Lobo AJ, et al. Indigo carmine-assisted high-magnification chromoscopic colonoscopy for the detection and characterization of intraepithelial neoplasia in ulcerative colitis: a prospective evaluation. Endoscopy 2005;37:1186–92.
32. Kiesslich R, Neurath M. Chromo- and magnifying endoscopy for colorectal lesions. Eur J Gastroenterol Hepatol 2005;17:793–801.
33. Nishiyama S, Oka S, Tanaka S, et al. Is it possible to discriminate between neoplastic and nonneoplastic lesions in ulcerative colitis by magnifying colonoscopy? Inflamm Bowel Dis 2014;20:508–13.
34. East JE, Suzuki N, von Herbay A, et al. Narrow band imaging with magnification for dysplasia detection and pit pattern assessment in ulcerative colitis surveillance: a case with multiple dysplasia associated lesions or masses. Gut 2006;55:1432–5.
35. Dekker E, van den Broek FJ, Reitsma JB, et al. Narrow-band imaging compared with conventional colonoscopy for the detection of dysplasia in patients with longstanding ulcerative colitis. Endoscopy 2007;39:216–21.
36. Matsumoto T, Kudo T, Jo Y, et al. Magnifying colonoscopy with narrow band imaging system for the diagnosis of dysplasia in ulcerative colitis: a pilot study. Gastrointest Endosc 2007;66:957–65.
37. Pellisé M, López-Cerón M, Rodríguez de Miguel C, et al. Narrow-band imaging as an alternative to chromoendoscopy for the detection of dysplasia in longstanding inflammatory bowel disease: a prospective, randomized, crossover study. Gastrointest Endosc 2011;74:840–8.
38. van den Broek FJ, Fockens P, van Eeden S, et al. Narrow-band imaging versus high-definition endoscopy for the diagnosis of neoplasia in ulcerative colitis. Endoscopy 2011;43:108–15.
39. Watanabe K, Sogawa M, Yamagami H, et al. Endoscopic differential diagnosis between ulcerative colitis-associated neoplasia and sporadic neoplasia in surveillance colonoscopy using narrow band imaging. Dig Endosc 2011;23:S143–9.
40. Bisschops R, Bessissow T, Baert F, et al. Chromo-endoscopy versus narrow band imaging in ulcerative colitis: a prospective randomized controlled trial. Endoscopy 2012;44:26.
41. Ignjatovic A, East JE, Subramanian V, et al. Narrow band imaging for detection of dysplasia in colitis: a randomized controlled trial. Am J Gastroenterol 2012;107:885–90.
42. Efthymiou M, Allen PB, Taylor AC, et al. Chromoendoscopy versus narrow band imaging for colonic surveillance in inflammatory bowel disease. Inflamm Bowel Dis 2013;19:2132–8.
43. Matsumoto T, Nakamura S, Moriyama T, et al. Autofluorescence imaging colonoscopy for the diagnosis of dysplasia in ulcerative colitis. Inflamm Bowel Dis 2007;13:640–1.

44. van den Broek FJ, Fockens P, van Eeden S, et al. Endoscopic tri-modal imaging for surveillance in ulcerative colitis: randomised comparison of high-resolution endoscopy and autofluorescence imaging for neoplasia detection; and evaluation of narrow-band imaging for classification of lesions. Gut 2008;57:1083–9.
45. Matsumoto T, Nakamura S, Moriyama T, et al. Autofluorescence imaging colonoscopy for the detection of dysplastic lesions in ulcerative colitis: a pilot study. Colorectal Dis 2010;12:291–7.
46. Soetikno R, Subramanian V, Kaltenbach T, et al. The detection of nonpolypoid (flat and depressed) colorectal neoplasms in patients with inflammatory bowel disease. Gastroenterology 2013;144:1349–52.
47. Wu L, Li P, Wu J, et al. The diagnostic accuracy of chromoendoscopy for dysplasia in ulcerative colitis: meta-analysis of six randomized controlled trials. Colorectal Dis 2012;14:416–20.
48. Tanaka S, Kaltenbach T, Chayama K, et al. High-magnification colonoscopy (with videos). Gastrointest Endosc 2006;64:604–13.
49. Sikka S, Ringold DA, Jonnalagadda S, et al. Comparison of white light and narrow band high definition images in predicting colon polyp histology, using standard colonoscopes without optical magnification. Endoscopy 2008;40:818–22.
50. Uraoka T, Saito Y, Matsuda T, et al. Detectability of colorectal neoplastic lesions using a narrow-band imaging system: a pilot study. J Gastroenterol Hepatol 2008;23:1810–5.
51. East JE, Suzuki N, Stavrinidis M, et al. Narrow band imaging for colonoscopic surveillance in hereditary non-polyposis colorectal cancer. Gut 2008;57:65–70.
52. East JE, Suzuki N, Saunders BP. Comparison of magnified pit pattern interpretation with narrow band imaging versus chromoendoscopy for diminutive colonic polyps: a pilot study. Gastrointest Endosc 2007;66:310–6.
53. Rastogi A, Bansal A, Wani S, et al. Narrow-band imaging colonoscopy – a pilot feasibility study for the detection of polyps and correlation of surface patterns with polyp histologic diagnosis. Gastrointest Endosc 2008;67:280–6.
54. Inoue T, Murano M, Murano N, et al. Comparative study of conventional colonoscopy and pan-colonic narrow-band imaging system in the detection of neoplastic colonic polyps: a randomized, controlled trial. J Gastroenterol 2008;43:45–50.
55. Hirata M, Tanaka S, Oka S, et al. Magnifying endoscopy with narrow band imaging for diagnosis of colorectal tumors. Gastrointest Endosc 2007;65:988–95.
56. Tischendorf JJ, Schirin-Sokhan R, Streetz K, et al. Value of magnifying endoscopy in classifying colorectal polyps based on vascular pattern. Endoscopy 2010;42:22–7.
57. Henry ZH, Yeaton P, Shami VM, et al. Meshed capillary vessels found on narrow-band imaging without optical magnification effectively identifies colorectal neoplasia: a North American validation of the Japanese experience. Gastrointest Endosc 2010;72:118–26.
58. Rastogi A, Pondugula K, Bansal A. Recognition of surface mucosal and vascular patterns of colon polyps by using narrow-band imaging: interobserver and intraobserver agreement and prediction of polyp histology. Gastrointest Endosc 2009;69:716–22.
59. Chiu HM, Chang CY, Chen CC, et al. A prospective comparative study of narrow-band imaging, chromoendoscopy, and conventional colonoscopy in the diagnosis of colorectal neoplasia. Gut 2007;56:373–9.
60. East JE, Suzuki N, Bassett P, et al. Narrow band imaging with magnification for the characterization of small and diminutive colonic polyps: pit pattern and vascular pattern intensity. Endoscopy 2008;40:811–7.

61. Sano Y, Ikematsu H, Fu KI, et al. Meshed capillary vessels by use of narrow-band imaging for differential diagnosis of small colorectal polyps. Gastrointest Endosc 2009;69:278–83.
62. Hüneburg R, Lammert F, Rabe C, et al. Chromocolonoscopy detects more adenomas than white light colonoscopy or narrow band imaging colonoscopy in hereditary nonpolyposis colorectal cancer screening. Endoscopy 2009;41: 316–22.
63. Rex DK, Helbig CC. High yields of small and flat adenomas with high-definition colonoscopes using either white light or narrow band imaging. Gastroenterology 2007;133:42–7.
64. Kaltenbach T, Friedland S, Soetikno R. A randomized tandem colonoscopy trial of narrow band imaging versus white light examination to compare neoplasia miss rates. Gut 2008;57:1406–12.
65. Adler A, Pohl H, Papanikolaou IS, et al. A prospective randomised study on narrow-band imaging versus conventional colonoscopy for adenoma detection: does narrow-band imaging induce a learning effect. Gut 2008;57:59–64.
66. Ikematsu H, Saito Y, Tanaka S, et al. The impact of narrow band imaging for colon polyp detection: a multicenter randomized controlled trial by tandem colonoscopy. J Gastroenterol 2012;47:1099–107.
67. Watanabe T, Ajioka Y, Matsumoto T, et al. Target biopsy or step biopsy? Optimal surveillance for ulcerative colitis: a Japanese nationwide randomized controlled trial. J Gastroenterol 2011;46:S11–6.

Implementation of Image-enhanced Endoscopy into Solo and Group Practices for Dysplasia Detection in Crohn's Disease and Ulcerative Colitis

 CrossMark

Rupert W. Leong, MD, FRACP[a], Rhys O. Butcher, MB ChB, MRCP[a],
Michael F. Picco, MD, PhD, FACG[b],*

KEYWORDS

- Ulcerative colitis • Crohn's colitis • Inflammatory bowel disease • Dysplasia
- Chromoendoscopy • Implementation

KEY POINTS

- Chromoendoscopy increases dysplasia detection in ulcerative colitis, and can be implemented across solo and group practices.
- Chromoendoscopy may not increase procedure time if the practice of random surveillance biopsies is abandoned.

INTRODUCTION

Image-enhanced colonoscopy using chromoendoscopy (CE) with targeted biopsy has been shown to significantly improve dysplasia detection in inflammatory bowel disease (IBD) colitis. However, the more commonly practiced method for dysplasia detection in ulcerative colitis (UC) and Crohn's colitis in the United States has historically included the low-yielding process of multiple randomly obtained mucosal biopsies.[1–3] White-light colonoscopy alone, without the aid of enhanced imaging or detailed inspection, is imperfect and lacks acceptable sensitivity and specificity,[4,5] with the yield of random biopsy for dysplasia ranging from 0% to 0.2%.[6–9]

Dysplasia detection rates are significantly higher with CE,[7,10] such that CE with targeted biopsy is now recommended.[1,2] Adopting the technique into clinical practice

Disclosure Statement: The authors have nothing to disclose.
[a] Gastroenterology and Liver Services, Concord Hospital, Sydney, Australia; [b] Division of Gastroenterology, Department of Medicine, Mayo Clinic, 4500 San Pablo Road, Jacksonville, FL 32224, USA
* Corresponding author.
E-mail address: picco.michael@mayo.edu

Gastrointest Endoscopy Clin N Am 24 (2014) 419–425
http://dx.doi.org/10.1016/j.giec.2014.04.001
1052-5157/14/$ – see front matter © 2014 Elsevier Inc. All rights reserved.

has been perceived to be difficult because of availability, lack of endoscopist experience, reliability of image interpretation, cost, and the additional time needed to perform the procedure. This article reviews the commonly available technique of CE. From our own experience and study, suggestions are provided of the key steps for the implementation of CE into solo and group clinical practices for UC dysplasia surveillance.

CE
The Technique

CE involves the application of dye solutions (indigo carmine or methylene blue) onto the colonic mucosa to enhance contrast during surveillance colonoscopy.[11] Studies showing significantly higher yield of dysplasia detection using CE compared with white-light colonoscopy have used both dyes, with concentrations range from 0.03% to 0.4% for adequate mucosal enhancement. Indigo carmine is a plant-based dye that pools into the mucosal crevices and can subsequently be washed away. Methylene blue is a vital dye that is actively taken up by the colonic epithelium after approximately 60 seconds.[11] It has been associated with DNA damage of unclear clinical significance.[12]

Adequate colonic preparation quality is essential when using CE. As such, during colonoscope insertion, irrigate the colon using water and simethicone, and suction any remaining debris. The washing of residue during intubation thoroughly cleans the mucosa before the application of CE, and in turn improves the overall efficiency of the procedure. Once the cecum is reached and the mucosa is cleaned, exchange the water irrigation bottle for the dye solution, and initiate dye spraying. The diluted dye can then be sprayed onto the mucosa using a standard flushing pump attached to the scope, either through pressing a foot pedal or a programmed button on the endoscope handle (**Fig. 1**). Direct the spray to the antigravity side of the colon in order to optimize the dye application to all of the colonic mucosa in an efficient manner. Other studies and practices use a spray catheter for dye application, whereby the

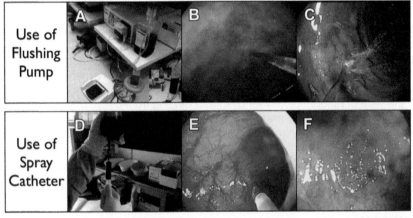

Fig. 1. Methods of application of CE. (*A*) Flushing pump with diluted CE solution in the irrigation bottle, and use of foot pump (*inset*). (*B*) CE spray onto colonic mucosa from the water channel can be seen during withdrawal. (*C*) During withdrawal, using CE, a nonpolypoid lesion is identified. (*D*) Preparation of diluted CE solution and transfer to syringes for spray catheter application. (*E*) Spray catheter is placed into the lumen and the CE solution is sprayed onto the mucosa during withdrawal (*F*).

endoscopist directs the catheter probe out of the endoscope accessory channel and the assistant continuously sprays the dye through the catheter using a 60-mL syringe while the endoscopist withdrawals the endoscope. The most recent descriptions and studies on CE using the flushing pump have shown it to be an efficient method of dye application because it eliminates the cost of the spray catheter as well as dependency on the assistant's spray catheter technique.

IMPLEMENTATION INTO PRACTICE

The implementation of CE with targeted biopsy for surveillance of dysplasia in patients with IBD requires emphasis on standardization of procedure, quality assurance, and training (**Table 1**).

Quality

The adoption of CE for UC dysplasia surveillance across solo and group practices requires the implementation of quality standards. Although the procedure is simple, its adequate performance requires acceptable dysplasia detection and procedure duration. Standardized procedures and reporting allow determination of minimal standards and the effect of CE on the development of colorectal cancer in UC. A transition period of combining targeted and random biopsy may be considered before abandoning random surveillance biopsies. Furthermore, it may be appropriate to identify 1 or a few endoscopists within a practice to perform the technique based on procedure volume, because outcomes may be improved with high volume.

In our study of 3 academic sites, we implemented the practice of CE for surveillance colonoscopy in patients with IBD initially through a research protocol.[13] We selected 6 gastroenterologists, who were not experts in IBD endoscopy, to participate. They reviewed the literature along with video examples as well as the practice protocol. Together, a pair of the participating endoscopists performed the initial procedures to review the technique and refine the protocol. There was eventual agreement on the CE technique using indigo carmine through the flushing pump. There was also agreement that any identified large lesion or one that would be technically difficulty to remove would be referred to an endoscopic resection expert within their group. We centrally recorded the procedure information.

Training

The issue of training is important. The American Gastroenterological Association recommends CE with targeted biopsy, provided that there is expertise available. However, CE is not taught during fellowship and there has never been by any effort to train. Therefore, in practice, CE is not performed in the United States. How should clinicians train when there is no trainer?

Familiarity with the detection of the nonpolypoid colorectal neoplasms is a prerequisite. The nonpolypoid neoplasms have been recognized in the United States only since 2008; again, most endoscopists did not have the opportunity to learn about detection, diagnosis, and treatment during fellowship. Given of the paucity of trainers, we suggest self-learning. Several learning videos are available, particularly through the American Society for Gastrointestinal Endoscopy (ASGE) Online Learning Library. Start by learning the detection of nonpolypoid neoplasms in patients who do not have IBD, as well as learning image-enhanced endoscopy. A training video on the use of CE with targeted biopsy is now available through the ASGE Online Learning Library. The published descriptions of the nonpolypoid colorectal neoplasms in colitic IBD can also provide printed guidance and an atlas for these efforts.

Table 1
Suggested steps for the implementation of CE into endoscopic practice

Equipment	
Colonoscope	High-definition colonoscope, monitor, and cables
Accessories	Apply chromoendoscopy via: Standard water pump attached to the endoscope activated via foot pedal Or: Dye-spray catheter • Length: 240 cm • Endoscope accessory channel: 2.8 mm Single-use spray catheters: • Olympus model PW-205V or Cook Medical Glo-Tip (GT-7-SPRAY) • Cost: AU$100–171 per catheter Reusable spray catheters: • Olympus model PW-5V-1 • Cost: AU$200 per catheter
Contrast agent	Indigo carmine (Sigma-Aldrich) • Cost: AU$37.80 per vial • Dilution: 0.5% (topical application) • For application via the foot pump, mix 2 vials of indigo carmine with 250 mL water (0.03%) Methylene blue (50 mg in 5 mL, Phebra) • Storage: <25°C • Cost: AU$36.00 per vial • Dilution: 0.1% (topical application)

Procedure and Protocol	
Time allotment	Consider initially during the learning curve period double colonoscopy time slot. Procedure times for CE have included random biopsies
Standard operating procedure	Complete colonoscopy to cecum • Lavage with water and suction during intubation Prepare contrast solution during insertion for application via the foot pump or spray • Indigo carmine: mix 2 vials of indigo carmine with 250 mL water (0.03%) • Indigo carmine: mix to indigo carmine with 1000cc water to obtain a concentration of 0.1 to 0.4% If using a foot pump: once the cecum is intubated, the water irrigation can be exchanged with the contrast solution. Apply the CE in a circumferential technique withdrawing the colonoscope If using a spray catheter: the dye-spray catheter is inserted into the working channel; the catheter tip should protrude 2–3 cm from the endoscope • Apply catheter dye solution segmentally using a rotational technique, withdrawing the colonoscope at the same time to cover the surface mucosa with dye Suction any excess solution after approximately 1 min to aid mucosal visualization • Focus on segments of 20–30 cm sequentially with reinsertion of the endoscope to the proximal extent of each segment before slow withdrawal and mucosal visualization Remove endoscopically resectable suspicious lesions using polypectomy or EMR Take targeted biopsies of any nonresectable abnormality visualized through CE to diagnose dysplasia Take biopsies of flat area surrounding lesions suspicious for dysplasia Consider tattoo of suspicious dysplastic lesion arising from flat mucosa or not able to be completely removed Take 2 random biopsies in every bowel segment to document microscopic disease activity

(continued on next page)

Table 1 (continued)	
Biopsies	
Circumscribed lesion	Biopsy of area surrounding lesion; lesions may be removed with polypectomy or EMR
Targeted and random biopsies	Targeted biopsies (can avoid random biopsies) of identified lesions in good-quality CE Segmental random biopsies for disease activity documentation
Training	
Trainees	Gastroenterology fellows and attendings
In-service training for nursing staff	Recommended
Trainer	Specialized endoscopist: training video is also available from the ASGE Learning Library to familiarize clinicians with the technique and the appearance of nonpolypoid colorectal neoplasms
Learning curve	Consider transition period of CE with targeted and random biopsy One study showed that endoscopists were partnered for the first 5 cases, and that procedure time plateaued at 15 cases
Learning environment and resources	Optimal setup of processor, monitor, and cables for optimal imaging Endoscopy software with image capture Endoscopy atlas Training videos Online resources Multidisciplinary meetings
Ease of learning	
Technical	Simple
Image recognition	Moderate
Quality Measures	
Selection of colitis cases based on accepted surveillance guidelines	Recommended
Colonoscopy quality measures	Recommended, such as bowel preparation quality, cecal intubation rating, withdrawal times, adenoma detection
Completeness of procedure (photographs)	Recommended photographs of terminal ileum, cecum, and any lesion; in addition, consider segmental photographic documentation even if no lesion seen
Review of images	Recommended study of images after examination, as well as after review of pathology
GI pathologist's verification	Recommended
Audit	Recommended (concordance with biopsies); additional quality indicators may include total procedural time, yield of targeted biopsies, volume of contrast agent

Abbreviations: ASGE, American Society for Gastrointestinal Endoscopy; EMR, endoscopic mucosal resection; GI, gastrointestinal.

In our CE implementation study, we assessed the feasibility of learning image interpretation. The 6 endoscopists underwent a short training session that consisted of viewing a teaching file of images and general instruction on the CE technique. Withdrawal times from the cecum and accuracy of image interpretation were measured.[13] Agreement of image interpretation was excellent for both white light and CE. Dysplasia detection rates were similar to published data from experts.

Procedure Time

The additional procedure time to perform CE is also a potential barrier to implementation. In a meta-analysis from experienced centers, CE increased procedure time by 11 minutes overall.[10] For patients who underwent tandem colonoscopies (the first under white light followed by indigo carmine staining), median extubation times were 11 minutes and 10 minutes respectively.[8] In another study, CE increased colonoscopy time from 35 to 44 minutes overall.[14] However, most of the reported times have also included the time taken for random biopsy. If the practice of random biopsies was abandoned in favor of targeted biopsies based on enhanced imaging, overall procedure time may be affected little and cost savings may be realized by restricting biopsies to targeted lesions.

In our implementation study, we also observed a learning curve with the technique. Withdrawal time decreased with experience, ranging from 31 minutes for fewer than 5 procedures to 19 minutes for more than 15 procedures completed.[13]

SUMMARY

CE with targeted colonic biopsies identifies dysplasia more readily than random biopsies and this evidence-based approach should therefore be adopted into group and solo practice.[1,2,15,16] The technique is easy and requires a low level of equipment. Mechanisms for its implementation include standardization of protocol and training, and ensuring quality metrics.

REFERENCES

1. Itzkowitz SH, Present DH, Crohn's and Colitis Foundation of America Colon Cancer in IBD Study Group. Consensus conference: colon cancer screening and surveillance in inflammatory bowel disease. Inflamm Bowel Dis 2005;11:314–21.
2. Farraye FA, Odze RD, Eaden J, et al. AGA technical review on the diagnosis and management of colorectal neoplasia in inflammatory bowel disease. Gastroenterology 2010;138:746–74.
3. Kornbluth A, Sachar DB. Ulcerative colitis practice guidelines in adults: American College of Gastroenterology Practice Parameters Committee. Am J Gastroenterol 2010;105:501–23.
4. Shanahan F, Quera R. CON: surveillance for ulcerative colitis-associated cancer: time to change the endoscopy and the microscopy. Am J Gastroenterol 2004;99: 1633–6.
5. Fujii S, Fujimori T, Chiba T, et al. Efficacy of surveillance and molecular markers for detection of ulcerative colitis-associated colorectal neoplasia. J Gastroenterol 2003;38:1117–25.
6. van den Broek F, Stokkers PC, Reitsma JB, et al. Random biopsies taken during colonoscopy surveillance of patients with longstanding ulcerative colitis; low yields and absence of clinical consequences. Am J Gastroenterol 2011;93:1–8.
7. Hurlstone DP, Sanders DS, Lobo AJ, et al. Indigo carmine-assisted high magnification chromoscopic colonoscopy for the detection and characterization of

intraepithelial neoplasia in ulcerative colitis: a prospective evaluation. Endoscopy 2005;37:1186–92.

8. Rutter MD, Saunders BP, Schofield G, et al. Pancolonic indigo carmine dye spraying for the detection of dysplasia in ulcerative colitis. Gut 2004;53:256–60.

9. Marion JF, Waye JD, Present DH, et al. Chromoendoscopy-targeted biopsies are superior to standard colonoscopic surveillance for detecting dysplasia in inflammatory bowel disease patients: a prospective endoscopic trial. Am J Gastroenterol 2008;103:2342–9.

10. Subramanian V, Mannath J, Ragunath K, et al. Meta-analysis: the diagnostic yield of chromoendoscopy for detecting dysplasia in patients with colonic inflammatory bowel disease. Aliment Pharmacol Ther 2011;33:304–12.

11. Kiesslich R, Neurath MF. Chromoendoscopy in inflammatory bowel disease. Gastroenterol Clin North Am 2012;41:291–302.

12. Oliver JR, Wild CP, Sahey P, et al. Chromoendoscopy with methylene blue and associated DNA damage in Barrett's oesophagus. Lancet 2003;362:373–4.

13. Picco MF, Pasha S, Leighton JA, et al. Procedure time and the determination of polypoid abnormalities with experience: implementation of a chromoendoscopy program for surveillance colonoscopy in ulcerative colitis. Inflamm Bowel Dis 2013;9:1913–20.

14. Kiesslich R, Fritsch J, Holtmann M, et al. Methylene blue-aided chromoendoscopy for the detection of intraepithelial neoplasia and colon cancer in ulcerative colitis. Gastroenterology 2003;124:880–8.

15. Cairns SR, Scholefield JH, Steele RJ, et al, British Society of Gastroenterology, Association of Coloproctology for Great Britain and Ireland. Guidelines for colorectal cancer screening and surveillance in moderate and high risk groups (update from 2002). Gut 2010;59:666–89.

16. Annese V, Daperno M, Rutter MD, et al, ECCO. European evidence based consensus for endoscopy in inflammatory bowel disease. J Crohns Colitis 2013;7:982–1018.

Beyond Standard Image-enhanced Endoscopy Confocal Endomicroscopy

Daniel Teubner, MD[a], Ralf Kiesslich, MD[a],*,
Takayuki Matsumoto, MD[b], Johannes W. Rey, MD[a],
Arthur Hoffman, MD[a]

KEYWORDS

- IBD • Confocal endomicroscopy • Chromoendoscopy

KEY POINTS

- Endomicroscopy is a new imaging tool for gastrointestinal endoscopy.
- Panchromoendoscopy with targeted biopsies has become the method of choice for surveillance of patients with inflammatory bowel disease.
- Endomicroscopy can be added after chromoendoscopy to clarify whether standard biopsies are still needed.
- This smart biopsy concept can increase the diagnostic yield of intraepithelial neoplasia and substantially reduce the need for biopsies.
- Endomicroscopy is still mainly used for research but clinical acceptance is increasing because of a multitude of positive studies about the diagnostic value of endomicroscopy.

INTRODUCTION

Patients with long-standing extensive chronic inflammatory bowel disease (IBD) have an increased risk to develop intraepithelial neoplasia and colitis-associated cancer compared with the average population risk. Triggers to neoplasia are chronic inflammation and sporadic adenoma.[1] Thus, colonoscopic surveillance is recommended in patients with long-lasting ulcerative colitis (left side and pancolitis) as well as Crohn's colitis.[2] Guidelines recommend performing targeted (visible lesions) and random biopsies. Here, 2 to 4 random biopsies every 10 cm within the colon should be performed.[2] Dysplastic lesions are often multifocal, flat, and difficult to detect with white light endoscopy.[2]

---

[a] Department for Internal Medicine, Gastroenterology and Oncology, St Marienkrankenhaus, Richard-Wagner-Street, 14, Frankfurt 60318, Germany; [b] Department of Medicine and Clinical Science, Graduate School of Medical Sciences, Kyushu University, Fukuoka, Japan
* Corresponding author.
E-mail address: info@ralf-kiesslich.de

Gastrointest Endoscopy Clin N Am 24 (2014) 427–434
http://dx.doi.org/10.1016/j.giec.2014.03.012
1052-5157/14/$ – see front matter © 2014 Elsevier Inc. All rights reserved.

In 2003, the first randomized controlled trial[3] was published evaluating lesions in the colon according to a modified pit pattern classification after panchromoendoscopy with methylene blue (0.1%) (pit pattern I–II, endoscopic prediction of nonneoplastic lesions; pit pattern III–V, endoscopic prediction of neoplastic lesions). Chromoendoscopy made it possible to identify dysplastic lesions and to clarify the borders between neoplastic and normal tissue. This development has led to the smart biopsy concept, in which more targeted biopsies become possible after enhanced endoscopy (chromoendoscopy) (**Figs. 1–3**). Panchromoendoscopy has become the method of choice for endoscopic surveillance of patients with IBD (European consensus guidelines).[2]

Confocal laser endomicroscopy (CLE) is a research and clinical tool that promises to improve diagnostics and therapeutic algorithms in patients with IBD. Endomicroscopy has been shown to be useful in dysplasia detection and differentiation of lesions to optimize their management (differentiation between colitis-associated neoplasia, sporadic neoplasia, and nonneoplastic lesions) and to reduce the number of unnecessary biopsies.[4] Confocal endomicroscopy has for the first time revealed in vivo tissue microscopy to gastroenterologists.[4] Using this technology, changes in vessel, connective tissue, and cellular-subcellular structures can be graduated during ongoing colonoscopy at subcellular resolution.[5,6]

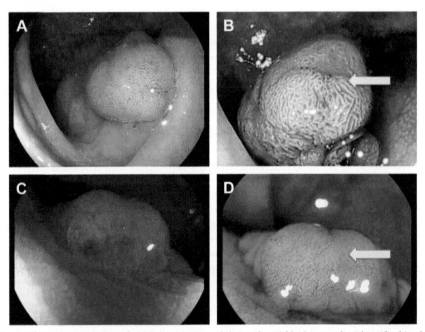

Fig. 1. Chromoendoscopy of colorectal lesions. (*A*) A polypoid lesion can be identified in the ascending colon of a 64-year-old patient who has had ulcerative colitis for 34 years. (*B*) Chromoendoscopy with methylene blue (0.1%) clarifies the mucosal pattern (pit pattern IIIL, *arrow*), which predicts tubular adenoma. Endoscopic resection was performed and final histology confirmed adenoma with low-grade intraepithelial neoplasia. (*C*) A sessile lesion can also be identified. A wide cryptal opening is seen (pit pattern II) using magnification and chromoendoscopy (*D*). Hyperplastic changes (nonneoplastic) could be confirmed histologically.

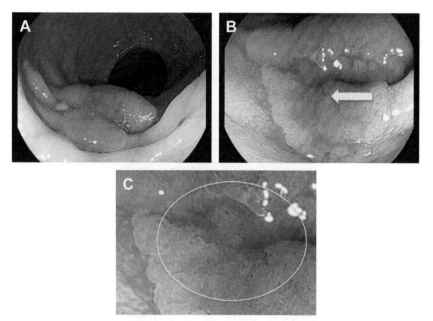

Fig. 2. Colitis-associated dysplasia. (*A*) A flat lesion is visible using white light high-definition colonoscopy. (*B*) Chromoendoscopy with methylene blue (0.1%) clarifies the borders and surface architecture. An irregular pattern with shallow depression (type IIc, pit pattern V) can be identified (*arrow* and magnified view [*C*]). Endoscopic resection revealed colitis-associated early cancer (shallow infiltration of the submucosal layer).

Confocal endomicroscopy has been shown to decrease the need for random biopsies because it has a high negative predictive value. Its use is often combined with chromoendoscopy. Intravital staining is used to identify lesions and targeted endomicroscopy is performed to clarify the need for standard biopsies. Thus, endomicroscopically normal-looking mucosa does not usually require further standard biopsies. Neoplastic changes and regenerative tissue can readily be identified using this method. However, detailed knowledge about the microarchitecture of the mucosa is necessary to achieve high diagnostic yields.[6,7]

TECHNICAL PRINCIPLES OF CONFOCAL ENDOMICROSCOPY

The CLE technique introduced in 2004 has been developed for cellular and subcellular imaging of the mucosal layer.[5] In confocal microscopy, a low-power laser is focused to a single point in a microscopic field of view and the same lens is used as both condenser and objective folding the optical path, so the point of illumination coincides with the point of detection within the specimen.[6] Light emanating from that point is focused through a pinhole to a detector and light emanating from outside the illuminated spot is not detected.

Because the illumination and detection systems are at the same focal plane, they are termed confocal.[6] All detected signals from the illuminated spot are captured and the created image is an optical section representing 1 focal plane within the examined specimen. The image of a scanned region can be constructed and digitized by measuring the light returning to the detector from successive points, and every point is typically scanned in a raster pattern.[6]

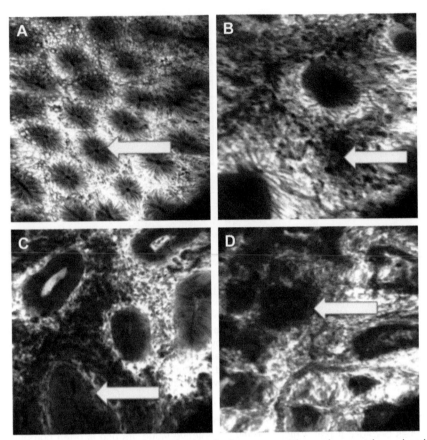

Fig. 3. Endomicroscopy in IBD. (*A*) Normal colonic mucosa with regular crypt (*arrow*) architecture can be seen. (*B*) Inflammatory cells can be identified within the lamina propria and are a sign of chronic inflammatory changes. (*C*) Inflammatory changes and dysplastic crypts (*arrow*) can be seen. The basement membrane is intact. Targeted biopsies confirmed the presence of low-grade intraepithelial neoplasia (colitis-associated dysplasia). (*D*) Colitis-associated cancer is present. Distorted glands with infiltration of malignant cells into the lamina propria (*arrow*) can be identified.

At present, 2 CLE-based systems are used in clinical routine and research (**Table 1**)[6,7]:

1. In CLE, a miniaturized confocal scanner is integrated into the distal tip of a flexible endoscope (Pentax Endomicroscopy System, Japan). A blue laser light source delivers an excitation wavelength of 488 nm, and light emission is detected at greater than 505 nm.[8] Successive points within the tissue are scanned in a raster pattern to construct serial en face optical section of 475 × 475 μm at a user-controlled variable imaging depth. Lateral resolution is 0.7 μm, and optical slice thickness is 7 μm (axial resolution). Images on the screen approximate a 1000-fold magnification of the tissue in vivo.[8]

2. The probe-based system (pCLE; Cellvizio Endomicroscopy System, Mauna Kea Technologies, Paris, France) consists of a 1.5-mm flexible miniprobe with lateral resolution between 3.5 μm and 1 μm, depending on the miniprobe, and axial resolution 5.0 μm. It is compatible with the working channel of any standard

Table 1
Technical aspects of endomicroscopic systems

	Endoscope Based	Probe Based
Outer diameter (mm)	12.8	1.0; 2.7; 2.6[a]
Length (cm)	120; 180	400; 300[a]
Field of view (μm)	475 × 475	320; 240; 600 μm[2a]
Resolution	0.7	3.5; 1.0[a]
Magnification	×1000	×1000
Imaging plane depth (μm)	0–250 (dynamic)	40–70; 55–65; 70–130 (fixed)[a]

[a] Dependent on various probes.

endoscope.[7,8] These probes can be fitted through the working channel of most endoscopes for clinical use. Image acquisition is faster with this probe (12 frames/s) at the expense of resolution being limited by the number of fibers (30,000 single fibers = pixels).

Compared with probe-based CLE, endoscopic CLE has slightly higher lateral resolution (approximately 0.7 vs 1.0 μm), a larger field of view (approximately 475 vs 240 μm), and variable imaging plane depth (approximately 0–250 vs 0–65 μm). However, the miniprobe is currently the only commercially available system and it can be used in conjunction with any standard endoscope. It is simply passed over the working channel and endomicroscopic images at video-frame rates are obtained, which allows a dynamic examination of the vessels and microarchitecture (12 vs 0.8–1.6 frames per second)/14).

Endomicroscopy requires contrast agents. The most commonly used dyes are fluorescein (intravenous application), acriflavine (local application), and cresyl violet (local application).[8–11]

The potential of endomicroscopy is not only in vivo histology. Endomicroscopy is also able to display and observe physiologic and pathophysiologic changes during ongoing endoscopy. Molecular imaging also becomes possible.[12] In inflammatory bowel diseases, CLE was able to spot intramucosal bacteria within the lamina propria.[13] These intramucosal bacteria are more common in patients with IBD compared with normal controls. These new visible details might refine understanding of IBD, because increased cell shedding is linked to increased amounts of intramucosal bacteria as well as a higher risk to develop a flare within 12 months.[14] Most recently endomicroscopy was used for molecular imaging; labeled antibodies (adalimumab) were applied topically onto the affected (inflamed) mucosa in patients with Crohn's disease. The number of membranous TNF-alpha receptors within the mucosa could be quantified and the response to biologic therapy could be predicted with high accuracy based on the fluorescence pattern of the receptors.[15]

CLINICAL TRIALS

An increasing body of literature has provided evidence that supports the concept of taking smart biopsies instead of untargeted, random specimens. Image-enhanced endoscopy using a dye-based technique (chromoendoscopy) and endomicroscopy are performed in combination. Chromoendoscopy provides the means for detection[16] with endomicroscopy for characterization.[17] The combination allows more neoplastic lesions to be detected and they can be differentiated from nonneoplastic lesions based on surface pattern architecture. Note that endomicroscopy of the whole gastrointestinal tract is not feasible because CLE has only a limited field of view (a maximum of 475–475 μm). The enhanced ability of chromoendoscopy and endomicroscopy to discriminate between nonneoplastic lesions, sporadic adenoma (adenomalike mass), and colitis-associated neoplasia (dysplasia-associated lesion masses) can potentially help to reduce the risk of colorectal cancer, lengthen surveillance intervals, and reduce the number of unnecessary biopsies (see **Fig. 3**).[2,3,15]

Panchromoendoscopy with either methylene blue or indigo carmine became a valid diagnostic tool for improving the diagnostic yield of intraepithelial neoplasia using the SURFACE guidelines in patients with IBD.[17] In the first randomized trial of endomicroscopy in ulcerative colitis, 153 patients with long-term ulcerative colitis who were in clinical remission were randomly assigned at a ratio of 1:1 to undergo either conventional colonoscopy or panchromoendoscopy using 0.1% methylene blue in conjunction with endomicroscopy to detect intraepithelial neoplasia or colorectal cancer.[4] Chromoendoscopy was used in this study to identify lesions for CLE and compared with standard white light endoscopy with random biopsies.

In vivo endomicroscopic prediction of the nature of lesions (neoplastic vs nonneoplastic) was accurate in 97.8% of lesions. In the conventional colonoscopy group, 42.2 biopsies were necessary. In the chromoendoscopy/CLE group, 3.9 biopsies per patient were sufficient, if only circumscribed lesions (by chromoendoscopy) with suspicious microarchitecture (by CLE) were biopsied.[4] The negative predictive value (NPV) for mucosa with a normal appearance on CLE to not harbor intraepithelial neoplasia was 99.1%, which reinforces the concept of taking smart biopsies instead of untargeted, random specimens.[4]

Sanduleanu and colleagues[18] showed that Acriflavine-guided endomicroscopy enables clinicians to differentiate between low-grade and high-grade intraepithelial neoplasia. Adenoma dysplasia score reliably discriminated high-grade dysplasia from low-grade dysplasia (accuracy, 96.7%). Interobserver agreement was high (K coefficients: pathologist, 0.92; endomicroscopist, 0.88). In vivo histology predicted ex vivo data with a sensitivity of 97.3%, specificity of 92.8%, and accuracy of 95.7%.

A meta-analysis of 91 studies, of which 11 on CLE by Wanders and colleagues[19] compared the pooled sensitivity, specificity, and real-time NPV of virtual chromoendoscopy (NBI, i-scan, FICE), CLE, and autofluorescence imaging for differentiation between neoplastic and nonneoplastic colonic lesions. This meta-analysis showed that virtual chromoendoscopy and CLE had an overall similar sensitivity and specificity, in that CLE produced the best results (sensitivity of 93% and specificity of 89%) and only CLE had a real-time NPV of more than 90%. A further meta-analysis of 15 studies of CLE, of which 4 on IBD by Su and colleagues[20] showed the effectiveness of CLE in discriminating between neoplastic and nonneoplastic lesions, showed similar results in pooled sensitivity and specificity, whereby specificity was even higher (sensitivity of 94% and specificity of 95%).

THE USE OF CRESYL VIOLET AND CONFOCAL ENDOMICROSCOPY

For tissue illumination with endomicroscopic low-power laser (488-nm blue laser light) application of fluorescence agents are necessary. Most studies in humans have been performed with intravenous fluorescein sodium (5 mL, 10%). Fluorescein quickly distributes within all compartments of the tissue, and CLE is possible within seconds after injection. It contrasts cellular and subcellular details, connective tissue, and vessel architecture at high resolution, but does not stain nuclei.[12]

Intravenous fluorescein is a nontoxic agent that is safe and mostly well tolerated, and only transient discoloration of the skin has been described.[12] CLE with intravenous fluorescein sodium allows analysis of cellular structure, connective tissue, and blood cells of the colonic mucosa in vivo. However, the nuclei of the intestinal epithelium are not readily visible because of the pharmacokinetic properties of fluorescein. Acriflavine and cresyl violet are alternative dyes that are applied topically and highlight nuclei, cell membranes, cytoplasm, and to a lesser extent vessels. Acriflavine accumulates in nuclei and therefore carries a potential mutagenic risk. Cresyl violet, which enriches in the cytoplasm and visualizes nuclear morphology negatively, is an alternative.

A 2-step study approach made in 2007 by Goetz and colleagues[21] evaluated the staining characteristics and optimal concentration of a single topical contrast agent, cresyl violet (Merck, Darmstadt, Germany) for simultaneous chromoendoscopy and CLE for straightforward and reliable recognition of lesions and their immediate characterization in vivo. After establishing the optimal cresyl violet dye concentration of 0.13% with a pH of 3.8 in an animal preclinical study, 67 sites in 36 patients in a prospective clinical study were topically stained and subsurface serial images were generated at different depths using CLE. The results showed a good resolution with chromoendoscopy for pit pattern classification and good fluorescent contrast for endomicroscopy. Imaging at variable penetration depths permitted high-resolution visualization of tissue architecture and subcellular details, such as mucin in goblet cells, and, more importantly, cell nuclei so that in vivo distinction of low-grade versus high-grade intraepithelial neoplasia was possible for the first time. Endomicroscopic targeting of biopsies to a region of altered nucleus/cytoplasm ratio on intravital staining with cresyl violet has resulted in the diagnosis of 1 additional case of high-grade intraepithelial neoplasia, and the overall prediction rate of neoplastic changes by CLE was excellent, although the small number of sites investigated may limit the significance of this finding.[21]

SUMMARY

Endomicroscopy is a new imaging tool for gastrointestinal endoscopy. In vivo histology becomes possible at subcellular resolution during ongoing colonoscopy.

Panchromoendoscopy with targeted biopsies has become the method of choice for surveillance of patients with IBD with IBD. Endomicroscopy can be added after chromoendoscopy to clarify whether standard biopsies are still needed. This smart biopsy concept can increase the diagnostic yield of intraepithelial neoplasia and substantially reduce the need for biopsies.

Endomicroscopy is still mainly used for research but clinical acceptance is increasing because of a multitude of positive studies about the diagnostic value of endomicroscopy. Different contrast agents are available to identify cellular and subcellular structures. Fluorescent agents can also be combined with proteins or antibodies to enable molecular imaging. Smart biopsies, functional imaging (eg, defining local barrier dysfunction), and molecular imaging (predicting the response to biologic therapy) may represent the future for endomicroscopy.

REFERENCES

1. Burisch J, Munkholm P. Inflammatory bowel disease epidemiology. Curr Opin Gastroenterol 2013;29(4):357–62.
2. Annese V, Daperno M, Rutter MD, et al. European evidence based consensus for endoscopy in inflammatory bowel disease. J Crohns Colitis 2013;7(12):982–1018.
3. Kiesslich R, Fritsch J, Holtmann M, et al. Methylene blue-aided chromoendoscopy for the detection of intraepithelial neoplasia and colon cancer in ulcerative colitis. Gastroenterology 2003;124:880–8.

4. Kiesslich R, Goetz M, Lammersdorf K, et al. Chromoscopy-guided endomicroscopy increases the diagnostic yield of intraepithelial neoplasia in ulcerative colitis. Gastroenterology 2007;132:874–82.

5. Kiesslich R, Burg J, Vieth M, et al. Confocal laser endoscopy for diagnosing intraepithelial neoplasias and colorectal cancer in vivo. Gastroenterology 2004; 127(3):706–13.

6. Goetz M, Watson A, Kiesslich R. Confocal laser endomicroscopy in gastrointestinal diseases. J Biophotonics 2011;4(7–8):498–508.

7. Liu J, Dlugosz A, Neumann H. Beyond white light endoscopy: the role of optical biopsy in inflammatory bowel disease. World J Gastroenterol 2013;19(43): 7544–5.

8. Neumann H, Kiesslich R, Wallace MB, et al. Confocal laser endomicroscopy: technical advances and clinical applications. Gastroenterology 2010;139(2): 388–92.

9. Kiesslich R, Canto MI. Confocal laser endomicroscopy. Gastrointest Endosc Clin N Am 2009;19(2):261–72.

10. Wallace MB, Meining A, Canto M, et al. The safety of intravenous fluorescein for confocal laser endomicroscopy in the gastrointestinal tract. Aliment Pharmacol Ther 2010;31(5):548–52.

11. Atreya R, Goetz M. Molecular imaging in gastroenterology. Nat Rev Gastroenterol Hepatol 2013;10(12):704–12.

12. Wang TD, Friedland S, Sahbaie P, et al. Functional imaging of colonic mucosa with a fibered confocal microscope for real-time in vivo pathology. Clin Gastroenterol Hepatol 2007;5(11):1300–5.

13. Moussata D, Goetz M, Gloeckner A, et al. Confocal laser endomicroscopy is a new imaging modality for recognition of intramucosal bacteria in inflammatory bowel disease in vivo. Gut 2011;60(1):26–33.

14. Kiesslich R, Duckworth CA, Moussata D, et al. Local barrier dysfunction identified by confocal laser endomicroscopy predicts relapse in inflammatory bowel disease. Gut 2012;61(8):1146–53.

15. Atreya R, Neumann H, Neufert C, et al. In vivo imaging using fluorescent antibodies to tumor necrosis factor predicts therapeutic response in Crohn's disease. Nat Med 2014;20(3):313–8.

16. Rutter MD, Saunders BP, Schofield G, et al. Pancolonic indigo carmine dye spraying for the detection of dysplasia in ulcerative colitis. Gut 2004;53:256–60.

17. Kiesslich R, Neurath MF. Surveillance colonoscopy in ulcerative colitis: magnifying chromoendoscopy in the spotlight. Gut 2004;53(2):165–7.

18. Sanduleanu S, Driessen A, Gomez-Garcia E, et al. In vivo diagnosis and classification of colorectal neoplasia by chromoendoscopy-guided confocal laser endomicroscopy. Clin Gastroenterol Hepatol 2010;8(4):371–8.

19. Wanders LK, East JE, Uitentuis SE, et al. Diagnostic performance of narrowed spectrum endoscopy, autofluorescence imaging, and confocal laser endomicroscopy for optical diagnosis of colonic polyps: a meta-analysis. Lancet Oncol 2013;14(13):1337–47.

20. Su P, Liu Y, Lin S, et al. Efficacy of confocal laser endomicroscopy for discriminating colorectal neoplasms from non-neoplasms: a systematic review and meta-analysis. Colorectal Dis 2013;15(1):e1–12.

21. Goetz M, Toermer T, Vieth M, et al. Simultaneous confocal laser endomicroscopy and chromoendoscopy with topical cresyl violet. Gastrointest Endosc 2009;70(5): 959–68.

Endoscopic Management of Nonpolypoid Colorectal Lesions in Colonic IBD

James E. East, MD(res), FRCP[a],*, Takashi Toyonaga, MD[b],
Noriko Suzuki, MD PhD[c]

KEYWORDS

- Colonoscopy • Colorectal cancer • Colitis • Colonic polyp • DALM • ALM
- Endoscopic mucosal resection • Endoscopic submucosal dissection

KEY POINTS

- Resection of nonpolypoid lesions in inflammatory bowel disease (IBD) is among the most technically demanding of endoscopic procedures.
- Inflammation and submucosal fibrosis make lesion preassessment and lifting difficult.
- En bloc excision is preferred where possible with snare or endoscopic submucosal dissection (ESD) to optimize the pathologic specimen and reduce recurrence risk.
- Close follow-up of the resection site and whole colon with dye-spray is required postresection.

Video of Endoscopic Submucosal Dissection (ESD) of a non-polypoid dysplastic lesion in ulcerative colitis accompanies this article at http://www.giendo. theclinics.com/

INTRODUCTION

The risk of developing IBD-colitis-related colorectal cancer has been highlighted for many years. Early data suggested that the risk increased year on year with an 18% risk at 30 years[1] and the initial British guidelines advocating shortening of surveillance intervals with each decade of disease.[2] Subsequent data suggested the stronger influence of patient factors, including disease extent and activity, family history of colorectal cancer, endoscopic features (strictures or postinflammatory polyps) and previous dysplasia, rather than duration of disease alone, with the current generation

[a] Translational Gastroenterology Unit, Experimental Medicine Division, Nuffield Department of Clinical Medicine, John Radcliffe Hospital, University of Oxford, Headley Way, Heading-ton, Oxford OX3 9DU, UK; [b] Department of Endoscopy, Kobe University Hospital, 7-5-1 Kusunoki-cho, Chou-ku, Kobe, Hyogo 650-0017, Japan; [c] Wolfson Unit for Endoscopy, St. Mark's Hospital, Watford road, Harrow, Middlesex HA1 3AY, UK
* Corresponding author.
E-mail address: jameseast6@yahoo.com

Gastrointest Endoscopy Clin N Am 24 (2014) 435–445
http://dx.doi.org/10.1016/j.giec.2014.03.003
1052-5157/14/$ – see front matter © 2014 Elsevier Inc. All rights reserved.

of European guidelines advocating risk-based stratification.[3–5] More recently, some population-based studies have suggested that previous results overestimate the risk of IBD dysplasia and cancer because of case selection from academic and tertiary centers.[6,7]

Alongside risk-based stratification, a new concept emerged for the management of polypoid dysplasia in IBD, in that polypoid circumscribed lesions (adenoma like masses) even within the colitic segment, might be safely managed by endoscopic resection and close follow-up rather than by panproctocolectomy.[4,5] A recent meta-analysis of 10 studies with more than 370 patients and 1700 years of patient follow-up supports this concept: 5 (95% confidence interval, 3–10) cancers developed per 1000 years of patient follow-up.[8] The rate of dysplasia detected at subsequent colonoscopy was 65 cases per 1000 years of patient follow-up, emphasizing that close colonoscopic surveillance is mandatory. However, all the studies in this meta-analysis predate the use of chromoendoscopy. The need for proctocolectomy when dysplasia is detected in IBD is based on older data, which suggested a 19% cancer rate at immediate proctocolectomy when low-grade dysplasia was detected and as much as 42% when high-grade dysplasia was found.[9] These data almost certainly related to a previous generation of endoscopes and endoscopists, the latter being less familiar than present-day endoscopists are with the appearances of nonpolypoid colorectal neoplasms, dysplasia, and cancer in IBD and hampered by a lack of high-quality endoscopic imaging. Furthermore, these endoscopists did not enjoy the advantages of high-definition, wide-angle endoscopes and dye-spray or image-enhanced endoscopy including structure enhancement, narrow-spectrum endoscopy (narrow band imaging [NBI, Olympus, Tokyo, Japan], Fujinon intelligent chromoendoscopy [FICE, Fujinon, Tokyo, Japan], i-Scan, image-enhanced endoscopy [Pentax, Tokyo, Japan]), autofluorescence, or confocal endomicroscopy (see the article on advanced imaging elsewhere in this issue). Therefore, dysplasia detected in the current era of endoscopes and endoscopists is likely to be at an early stage and can be safely managed by endoscopic resection if polypoid and circumscribed.

However, not all dysplasia detected at endoscopy in IBD is polypoid. The concept of flat dysplasia or endoscopically invisible dysplasia, detectable only by random biopsies has been commonly accepted, particularly in the prechromoendoscopy era, leading to previous generations of guidelines advocating the use of quadratic biopsies every 10 cm of colonoscopic withdrawal to detect this invisible dysplasia. This recommendation is poor for detection of early dysplasia, with one simulation paper based on colonic surface areas and dysplasia size suggesting that the standard 32 nontargeted biopsies would only detect an area of dysplasia encompassing 5% or more of the colonic surface with 80% certainty.[10] The use of the word flat for biopsy-only-detected dysplasia is unfortunate because this word has also been used to describe nonpolypoid dysplasia in the endoscopic literature as part of the Paris classification.[11] Flat or nonpolypoid in the endoscopic literature corresponds to Paris 0-IIa, flat elevated lesion; Paris 0-IIb, completely flat lesions; and Paris 0-IIc, depressed lesions. Many instances of patients diagnosed with flat biopsy-only dysplasia can be converted to circumscribed areas of dysplasia described as Paris 0-IIa, IIb, or IIc by reexamination with meticulous bowel preparation, with the patient in full remission, with an experienced endoscopist familiar with dysplasia in IBD, and with the use of high-definition endoscopes with dye-spray and image enhancement. If one accepts that circumscribed areas of flat dysplasia may be safely endoscopically resected with close endoscopic surveillance afterward,[12] a concept that is by no means proven, then one needs to consider the special circumstances of how to safely and comprehensively resect such lesions. The technique for endoscopic resection is the focus of this review.

APPROACH TO RESECT NONPOLYPOID DYSPLASIA IN IBD

The resection of mucosal dysplasia in the gastrointestinal tract requires a series of steps to be safe and effective, which are outlined in **Box 1**. Here, it is assumed that an isolated, ie, nonmultifocal, nonpolypoid (Paris 0-IIa, 0-IIb, or 0-IIc), lesion within a colitic segment has been detected; that the patient's case has been discussed at an IBD multidisciplinary team meeting with a recommendation for attempt at endoscopic resection; and that the patient, having discussed the pros and cons of an endoscopic approach and being informed of the risks and benefits, is willing to proceed. Furthermore, it is also assumed that as far as possible the patient is in remission from colitis and that the bowel is optimally prepared. Data on approach to these lesions are scarce and predominantly based on expert end consensus opinion, extrapolation from first principles, and from experiences with resection of dysplastic lesion in noncolitic colons in situations that may mimic colitis-related fibrosis, such as scarring from previous endoscopic resection or nongranular-type laterally spreading tumors (LSTs). By definition, endoscopic resection of dysplasia in colitis is at the far end of the spectrum of difficulty of endoscopic resection and should only be attempted by experienced, usually specialist endoscopists, with appropriate experience of advanced endoscopic mucosal resection (EMR), case volume, and an

---

Box 1
Approach to resect nonpolypoid dysplasia in IBD

- Lesion assessment
  - Extent
  - Risk of invasion
  - Associated structures, eg, ileocecal valve
  - Scarring
  - Endoscopic access
- Lifting
  - Mucosal inflammation/scarring
  - Special lift solution, eg, hyaluronate
- Resection
  - Endoscopic mucosal resection
    - En bloc
    - Piecemeal
  - Endoscopic submucosal dissection
  - Special snares (spiral or flat band/ribbon)
- Ablation
  - Argon plasma coagulation
  - Snare tip soft coagulation
- Follow-up
  - Scar assessment

endoscopic support team with surgical backup. Such cases might usually be referred to tertiary or regional specialists.

Lesion Assessment

A nonpolypoid dysplastic lesion in IBD needs to first be carefully examined. Thus, before considering an attempt at endoscopic resection and weighing the associated technical risks of bleeding, perforation, and postpolypectomy syndrome, as well as the ensuing risk of cancer within the resection specimen and recurrence, the lesion characteristics must be interpreted. The first question to be addressed is lesion borders and extent. Endoscopic resection is only appropriate for lesions that have clearly defined borders (ie, circumscribed). Enhancement of the edges of these subtle lesions can be helped by the use of dye-spray or advanced imaging techniques. If a clear margin of the lesion cannot be seen, it is unlikely that endoscopic resection is appropriate because there is significant risk that residual dysplasia will be left in situ (**Fig. 1**). Even if a clear border can be seen, it is appropriate to perform biopsies around the lesion to look for endoscopically invisible dysplasia before committing to resection. Ideally, only a single biopsy of the lesion itself would be done to avoid welding the lesion to the submucosa even further through biopsy-associated fibrosis. The authors' personal preference is to use a high-definition endoscope, ideally with optical magnification, and chromoendoscopy and surface enhancement for this process.

Assuming the lesion has a clear edge with no surrounding dysplasia on biopsy of macroscopically normal mucosa, the lesion should be completely clear of stool and mucus and minutely examined for risks of invasion. Suspicious aspects include a large nodule, depression and loss of pit pattern, and a masslike appearance (**Fig. 2**).[13] The presence of any of these signs should lead to a careful consideration of whether endoscopic resection is appropriate. Unfortunately, these techniques, which are reasonably reliable in noncolitic colons, perform less well in colitis, because the scarring may lead to pseudodepression and inflammation distorts pit patterns. The nonlifting sign, which in combination with macroscopic appearance gives a good estimate of likely invasion in the assessment of noncolitis-associated lesions, is by definition poor in colitis. Submucosal scarring impedes mucosal lift[14] and also disrupts the mucosal layers needed to clearly assess invasion at endoscopic ultrasonography. In noncolitis cases, submucosal scarring can be seen in lesions with a previous attempt at resection, recurrence on a scar from previous EMR, or nongranular type LSTs.[15] In

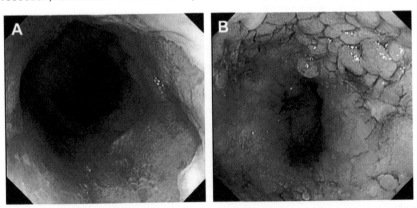

Fig. 1. This endoscopic image shows a nonpolypoid flat dysplastic area in the lower region of rectum (*A*). Despite use of dye-spray, a clearly circumscribed boarder cannot be delineated (*B*). Therefore, this lesion is not suitable for endoscopic resection.

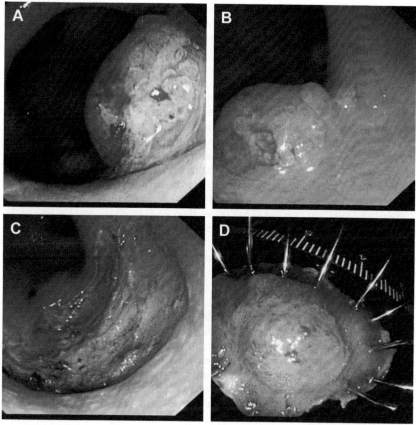

Fig. 2. This 15-mm lesion in the rectum of a 71-year-old woman with ulcerative colitis was selected for ESD. Note that the pit pattern is difficult to interpret and that it suggests a nodule or mass lesion (Paris 0-Is component), raising suspicion for invasion (*A, B*). En bloc excision was achieved with ESD; the histology showed early invasion (Kikuchi stage sm1) (*C, D*).

colitis cases, if the patient has a tubular colon with evidence of scarring, postinflammatory polyps, loss of vascular pattern, or active inflammation, the submucosal scarring is likely to be severe and typically involves the entire lesion.

Location of the lesion near technically difficult areas such as the appendix orifice, ileocecal valve, at a flexure, especially on the inside of the bend, and at the anal verge should also be considered.[16] Although polyps in all these positions can be resected in noncolitic colon by experienced endoscopists, the technical difficulty is substantially increased. In combination with the other inherent challenges that colitic lesions present, this may make the likelihood of a successful resection so low that an endoscopic attempt is not appropriate.

The final stage is to consider endoscopic access. This is one of the few areas in which working in a colitic colon may have advantages because a scarred and tubular colon makes for a straight endoscope and associated accurate tip movements and a lack of haustral folds to be negotiated. Before starting, endoscopists should be satisfied that they can easily reach all areas of the lesion with submillimeter precision.

There is no specific combination of factors or scoring system that suggests that lesions are or are not safely and effectively resectable. Ultimately, at least at present, it comes down to the experience and judgment of the assessing endoscopist. Given the fine nature of these judgments, the authors recommend that if possible the endoscopist who is going to do the resection procedure should perform the endoscopy for lesion assessment before resection.

Lifting

Lifting or the failure of lifting of lesions in colitis is one of the major obstacles to resection. This leads to problems with lesion assessment for invasion as outlined above, but more importantly means that the lesion cannot be safely lifted away from the underlying muscularis propria to allow a safe plane for the snare or endoscopic knife to traverse for resection. The scarring in the submucosa means that there is difficulty in finding the submucosal plane, a failure to lift, a 'diffuse' lift in which fluid tracks laterally rather than resulting in focal elevation, and a rapid loss of any lift achieved. Techniques to counter these problem include the use of the dynamic injection technique,[17] the use of thinner-bore injection needles (25 G rather than 21 G or 23 G), and the use of more viscous and longer-lasting injection solutions including colloids, eg, gelofusine,[18] or sodium hyaluronate.[19] Other viscous solutions, eg, hypromellose or glycerol, might also be considered.[19] Nevertheless, even with these advantages, lift in colitic lesions is often suboptimal.

Resection

En bloc resection of the lesion is preferable to allow precise pathologic assessment and minimize residual dysplasia or recurrence. ESD offers this possibility and is technically possible in colitis. However, the comprehensive submucosal fibrosis increases the procedural risks and reduces R0 resection rates even for superspecialist experts in ESD (**Figs. 3** and **4**). Use of small-caliber-tip transparent hoods can help in severe fibrosis, and there is often a need to use sharp-tipped needle knives to cut fibrotic bands, albeit at the risk of a loss of hemostatic capacity (Video 1).[20]

The adaptation of ESD concepts may offer some advantages to less-experienced Western endoscopists. Two concepts may be helpful.[21] The first is the so-called Endoscopic Mucosal Resection with snaretip incision (SI) that can be possible for smaller lesions up to 20 mm in which submucosal scarring is not so severe and some lift is possible. Here, after lifting, the snare tip is used to make a small incision on the oral side of the lesion. This small hole is used to anchor the snare tip to allow definite edge capture and additional downward pressure with the snare in a situation of limited lift, increasing the chances on an en bloc snare resection. The second is the use of mucosal incision, the first step in full ESD.[21] Here the use of an endoknife to carefully incise a groove around the lesion is performed before an attempt at conventional en bloc or piecemeal EMR. The edge of the snare is then placed in this marginal groove for resection. Both these concepts improve grip on the lesion edge by the snare and allow a clean resection margin at the edge of the lesion. In colitis, once resection starts, the lesion margin can be difficult to see, so marginal incision can assist here as well. This procedure is sometimes described as simplified or hybrid ESD and in some situations represents a good compromise between the time, risk, and difficulty of full ESD, yet fulfills the need for resection with a clear margin.

Snares

Standard snares can be used for EMR in colitis; however, as alluded to above, scarred, flat lesions with poor lift can be difficult to engage into the snare. Furthermore, if a large piece is successfully engaged, there is a risk that the scarring will pull up an area of underlying muscle leading to damage to the muscularis propria target sign or a

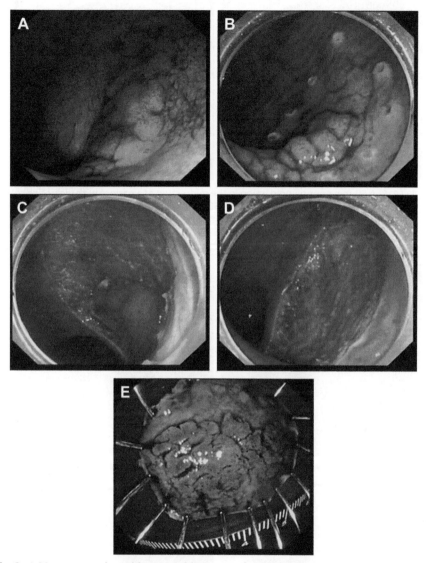

Fig. 3. A 20-mm nonpolypoid (Paris 0-IIa) lesion was found in the midrectum of a 53-year-old patient, with circumscribed edges after dye-spray (*A*). Marking was used to define the lesion edges clearly before mucosal incision. Although commonly used in ESD in the upper gastrointestinal tract, marking is rare in the colon; however, because of the subtle edges of the lesion, this may be helpful in colitis (*B*). A formal ESD is performed with en bloc excision (*C*, *D*) with the resected specimen showing clear margins (*E*). Pathology confirmed low-grade dysplasia.

full-thickness perforation.[22] Perforations are especially difficult to close in scarred mucosa. Braided or spiral snares may be used, which have an additional spiral wire around the main snare cable, to improve gripping (spiral snare 20 mm, SnareMaster, Olympus, Tokyo, Japan). An alternative is the flat band or ribbon snare (flat ribbon snare 22 m, Resection Master, Medwork, Höchstadt, Germany). This snare comprises

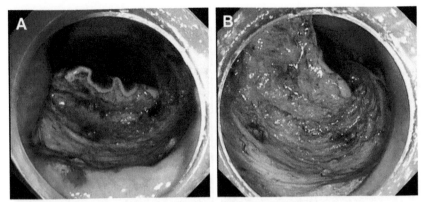

Fig. 4. (*A, B*) A 50-mm nonpolypoid lesion in the midrectum of a patient with ulcerative colitis was scheduled for an attempt at resection by ESD. Intense fibrosis was observed in the submucosal layer (yellow-white band under mucosal flap) making resection very challenging.

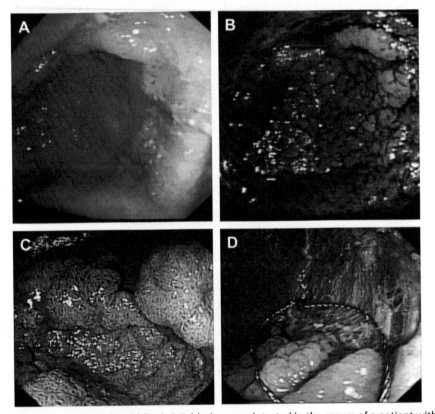

Fig. 5. A 35-mm nonpolypoid (Paris 0-IIa) lesion was detected in the cecum of a patient with long-standing pancolonic IBD (*A*). Use of dye-spray confirms a circumscribed lesion without high-risk features (*B*). Narrow band imaging is used to assess the microvessel network (*C*). The lesion is resected in 4 fragments by piecemeal EMR with a 10-mm snare (*D*). All fragments are retrieved with a Roth net for pathology assessment (*E*). Pathology confirms a tubulovillous adenoma with low-grade dysplasia (*F*) (Hematoxylin and eosin, original magnification ×400). Reassessment of the scar after healing with dye-spray showed no dysplasia either macroscopically or in scar biopsies (*G*).

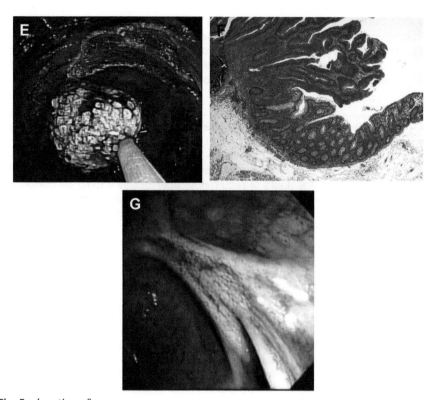

Fig. 5. (*continued*)

a flat band of metal to make the snare loop with the edge of the band orientated verti-
cally to the mucosa. An alternative is to use a smaller braided snare to resect small
pieces at a time, reducing the risk that too much mucosa is gathered with associated
muscle, as one might do for a scarred lesion in noncolitic colons (**Fig. 5**). A final option
is the use of a double-channel endoscope using a grasper to pull the mucosa into a
snare, which is in the other channel. Although this technique guarantees the ability
to grip the mucosa, the risk of perforation is significantly magnified, and experience
and extreme care are needed.

Ablation

Owing to the scarring in colitis, the nature of resection of colitic lesions often entails
piecemeal resection. Every attempt should be made to endoscopically resect any
visible part of the lesion. However, piecemeal resection coupled with significant
scaring may result in fragments or islands of dysplasia left at the resection site.
Such areas need to be definitively but safely destroyed. Argon plasma coagulation
(APC) has been commonly used for this with some evidence from the EMR literature
that it is effective in reducing recurrence.[23] (Many EMR experts suggest that the
need for this in noncolitic colons is now unnecessary because the EMR technique
has improved; however, older, less-comprehensive EMR to some extent mimics the
results in colitis so the two may be comparable.) Precise use of short pulses of APC
is effective even for larger areas. Further attempts at injection before use of APC

may allow the so-called melt effect seen with the use of APC for dysplasia ablation in the duodenum.[24] For small fragments, the use of the tip of the snare with soft coagulation allows effective ablation without overdelivery of energy and risks of a deep mucosal burn. Ultimately, the optimum is en bloc R0 snare or ESD resection with pathologic assessment of resected tissue. Ablation should be minimized.

Follow-Up

After resection, which should be as complete as possible at the first attempt, careful examination of the scar should be performed at between 2 and 6 months postresection, as well as pancolonic dye-spray of the whole colon to look for metachronous lesions. The use of dye-spray and advanced imaging on the scar can be helpful here to try and detect tiny areas of recurrence. Scar biopsy should be performed even if there is no recurrence. If recurrence is suspected, and the threshold should be low, a biopsy of the site followed by the ablation methods mentioned above is appropriate, with a further examination in 2 to 6 months. Repeated recurrence despite appropriate ablation, high-grade dysplasia in recurrence biopsies, or a large area of recurrence should prompt consideration of surgical resection or ESD salvage.

SUMMARY

Safe and comprehensive resection of nonpolypoid dysplasia in IBD is demanding both in terms of diagnostic judgments preresection and of technical skills during the resection. Good outcomes require meticulous planning and maximizing potential technical advantages, with an aim to achieve en bloc excision where possible. The safe resection of circumscribed nonpolypoid dysplasia in IBD is possible by an appropriately trained endoscopic team and may avoid the need for colectomy.

SUPPLEMENTARY DATA

Video related to this article can be found online at http://dx.doi.org/10.1016/j.giec.2014.03.003.

REFERENCES

1. Eaden JA, Abrams KR, Mayberry JF. The risk of colorectal cancer in ulcerative colitis: a meta-analysis. Gut 2001;48:526–35.
2. Eaden JA, Mayberry JF. Guidelines for screening and surveillance of asymptomatic colorectal cancer in patients with inflammatory bowel disease. Gut 2002;51:V10–2.
3. Colonoscopic surveillance for prevention of colorectal cancer in people with ulcerative colitis, Crohn's disease or adenomas: NICE guideline. Available at: http://www.nice.org.uk/nicemedia/live/13415/57930/57930.pdf. Accessed February 8, 2014.
4. Cairns SR, Scholefield JH, Steele RJ, et al. Guidelines for colorectal cancer screening and surveillance in moderate and high risk groups (update from 2002). Gut 2010;59:666–89.
5. Annese V, Daperno M, Rutter MD, et al. European evidence based consensus for endoscopy in inflammatory bowel disease. J Crohns Colitis 2013;7:982–1018.
6. Herrinton LJ, Liu L, Levin TR, et al. Incidence and mortality of colorectal adenocarcinoma in persons with inflammatory bowel disease from 1998 to 2010. Gastroenterology 2012;143:382–9.

7. Jess T, Simonsen J, Jorgensen KT, et al. Decreasing risk of colorectal cancer in patients with inflammatory bowel disease over 30 years. Gastroenterology 2012; 143:375–81.

8. Wanders LK, Dekker E, Pullens B, et al. Cancer risk after resection of polypoid dysplasia in patients with longstanding ulcerative colitis: a meta-analysis. Clin Gastroenterol Hepatol 2014;12:756–64.

9. Bernstein CN, Shanahan F, Weinstein WM. Are we telling patients the truth about surveillance colonoscopy in ulcerative colitis? Lancet 1994;343:71–4.

10. Awais D, Siegel CA, Higgins PD. Modelling dysplasia detection in ulcerative colitis: clinical implications of surveillance intensity. Gut 2009;58:1498–503.

11. Participants in the Paris Workshop. The Paris endoscopic classification of superficial neoplastic lesions: esophagus, stomach, and colon: November 30 to December 1, 2002. Gastrointest Endosc 2003;58:S3–43.

12. Hurlstone DP, Sanders DS, Atkinson R, et al. Endoscopic mucosal resection for flat neoplasia in chronic ulcerative colitis: can we change the endoscopic management paradigm? Gut 2007;56:838–46.

13. Uraoka T, Saito Y, Matsuda T, et al. Endoscopic indications for endoscopic mucosal resection of laterally spreading tumours in the colorectum. Gut 2006; 55:1592–7.

14. Uno Y, Munakata A. The non-lifting sign of invasive colon cancer. Gastrointest Endosc 1994;40:485–9.

15. Toyonaga T, Man-i M, Fujita T, et al. Retrospective study of technical aspects and complications of endoscopic submucosal dissection for laterally spreading tumors of the colorectum. Endoscopy 2010;42:714–22.

16. Moss A, Bourke MJ, Williams SJ, et al. Endoscopic mucosal resection outcomes and prediction of submucosal cancer from advanced colonic mucosal neoplasia. Gastroenterology 2011;140:1909–18.

17. Soetikno R, Kaltenbach T. Dynamic submucosal injection technique. Gastrointest Endosc Clin N Am 2010;20:497–502.

18. Moss A, Bourke MJ, Kwan V, et al. Succinylated gelatin substantially increases en bloc resection size in colonic EMR: a randomized, blinded trial in a porcine model. Gastrointest Endosc 2010;71:589–95.

19. Polymeros D, Kotsalidis G, Triantafyllou K, et al. Comparative performance of novel solutions for submucosal injection in porcine stomachs: an ex vivo study. Dig Liver Dis 2010;42:226–9.

20. Toyonaga T, Man I, Fujita T, et al. The performance of a novel ball-tipped Flush knife for endoscopic submucosal dissection: a case-control study. Aliment Pharmacol Ther 2010;32:908–15.

21. Toyonaga T, Man I, Morita Y, et al. The new resources of treatment for early stage colorectal tumors: EMR with small incision and simplified endoscopic submucosal dissection. Dig Endosc 2009;21(Suppl 1):S31–7.

22. Swan MP, Bourke MJ, Moss A, et al. The target sign: an endoscopic marker for the resection of the muscularis propria and potential perforation during colonic endoscopic mucosal resection. Gastrointest Endosc 2011;73:79–85.

23. Brooker JC, Saunders BP, Shah SG, et al. Treatment with argon plasma coagulation reduces recurrence after piecemeal resection of large sessile colonic polyps: a randomized trial and recommendations. Gastrointest Endosc 2002;55:371–5.

24. Tsiamoulos ZP, Peake ST, Bourikas LA, et al. Endoscopic mucosal ablation: a novel technique for a giant nonampullary duodenal adenoma. Endoscopy 2013;45(Suppl 2 UCTN):E12–3.

Surgical Management of Nonpolypoid Colorectal Lesions and Strictures in Colonic Inflammatory Bowel Disease

CrossMark

Lisa C. Coviello, DO[a],*, Sharon L. Stein, MD[b]

KEYWORDS

- Colorectal cancer • Inflammatory bowel disease • Dysplasia
- Nonpolypoid colorectal neoplasm • Stricture • Ulcerative colitis • Crohn's disease

KEY POINTS

- Patients with inflammatory bowel disease and dysplasia have pathologic characteristics and risks that differ from those of patients with sporadic carcinomas.
- Surgical interventions need to be more aggressive than in sporadic cases.
- An algorithm for management strategies for lesions and strictures in Crohn's disease and ulcerative colitis needs to be developed.
- A better understanding of the risks and benefits of surgical procedures for dysplasia in Crohn's disease and ulcerative colitis is required.

BACKGROUND

Colorectal cancer (CRC) arising in inflammatory bowel disease (IBD) accounts for only 1% to 2% of all general CRC cases per year. However, as CRC results in 15% of all IBD deaths, cancer screening requires special vigilance in this group. Particularly concerning is the fact that cancers in patients with ulcerative colitis and Crohn's disease often present not as mass lesions but as dysplasia, strictures, or diffuse dysplasia.

The risk of CRC in ulcerative colitis (UC) has been well studied. Most reliable risk factors associated with an increased risk of CRC in UC are related to the extent and duration of the disease. The risk for CRC development is lower before 8 to 10 years after onset of symptoms (3%); however, thereafter the risk increases by approximately

Relationships: None.
[a] Colorectal Surgery and Endoscopy, Department of Surgery, William Beaumont Army Medical Center, 5005 North Piedras Street, El Paso, TX 79920, USA; [b] Section of Colon and Rectal Surgery, Department of Surgery, University Hospitals/Case Medical Center, 11100 Euclid Avenue, LKS 5047, Cleveland, OH 44106, USA
* Corresponding author.
E-mail address: lccovi@gmail.com

Gastrointest Endoscopy Clin N Am 24 (2014) 447–454
http://dx.doi.org/10.1016/j.giec.2014.04.002
1052-5157/14/$ – see front matter Published by Elsevier Inc.

1% per year. Various studies have shown risks of CRC in UC ranging from 5% to 20% at 20 years of the disease.[1–3] By the fourth decade of UC disease, the risk of developing CRC is as high as 56 times higher than that of the general population.[4] In 2012, a large Danish population-based study demonstrated decreasing rates of CRC in UC over the last 30 years. This decrease is due possibly to the improved medical treatment of the disease in addition to surveillance of dysplasia.[5]

The rates of CRC in Crohn's disease seem to mirror those of UC.[6,7] Crohn's patients have a 5- to 20-fold increase in risk for CRC in comparison with the general population.[7,8] The absolute cumulative frequencies of CRC after 20 years of disease in both UC and Crohn's disease are similar at 8% and 7%, respectively.[9] Because of this similarity, despite the publication of fewer data regarding CRC in Crohn's disease, guidelines and recommendations have been developed for Crohn's patients extrapolating from the body of evidence on UC.

DYSPLASIA AS A PREDICTOR

The mutation pathway to CRC in IBD is postulated to be distinct from the adenoma-carcinoma sequence seen in sporadic colon cancers. Duration and extent of disease are both associated with higher rates of dysplasia and malignancy. IBD-associated cancer often develops in younger patients, and is more likely to be diffuse, extensive, multifocal, and mucinous, compared with the population with sporadic colorectal cancer.[10–12] Cancer in Crohn's disease is more likely to be right-sided and associated with ileal/right-sided inflammation.[9]

Furthermore, IBD patients with colon cancer have historically been shown to have synchronous dysplasia at distant sites from the cancer, suggesting the potential for a field defect rather than an isolated mutation. A review from more than 2 decades ago that included 10 prospective studies with a total of 1225 UC patients demonstrated cancer in 43% of patients with biopsy-proven high-grade dysplasia (HGD). Nineteen percent of patients with low-grade dysplasia (LGD) also had a coexistent cancer.[13] Dysplasia distant to the primary carcinoma has also been shown in 23% to 70% of patients with Crohn's disease.[8] Indeed, the reported risks of synchronous lesions have been variable, as high as 71% for synchronous dysplasia and ranging from 17% to 43% for synchronous cancers.[13–19]

Interpretation of the data on synchronous cancers should, however, be made with caution, owing to the significant limitations during that era in the sensitivity of the fiberoptic technology in detecting dysplasia or cancer at index colonoscopy. Furthermore, surveillance of patients with dysplasia was not standardized (eg, performed without chromoendoscopy or image enhancement at various intervals, or in the endoscopic removal techniques). The true incidence of synchronous colorectal cancer in the setting of dysplasia, as well as the true natural history of endoscopically invisible dysplasia, is thus not known.

For high-risk patients the decision regarding whether to proceed with colectomy or local endoscopic removal with continued colonoscopic surveillance is unquestionably complex, and requires a multidisciplinary approach.

DYSPLASIA MANAGEMENT
Endoscopically Visible Dysplasia

Nowadays most IBD-related dysplasia visible, following the advancements of endoscopic imaging and techniques and a deeper understanding of its appearance, and can be removed endoscopically. Furthermore, terminology for neoplasia in IBD is now being standardized to be similar to neoplasia not related to IBD (ie, polypoid and nonpolypoid for shape; and endoscopically resectable and endoscopically nonresectable for management). Historical terms such as adenoma-like dysplasia-associated lesion or mass (DALM) and non–adenoma-like DALM, or flat dysplasia, are being abandoned because they are regarded as confusing, and conceived when dysplasia was largely thought to be invisible during an era of lower-quality endoscopic imaging and interpretation.

In fact, longitudinal studies show that isolated adenomatous polyps may be safely removed endoscopically with close follow-up, analogous to sporadic adenoma removal in the absence of colitis. Such adenomatous polyps treated with endoscopic resection alone have been found to have no increased risk for cancer, as long as there is no evidence of dysplasia in the mucosa surrounding the polyp or elsewhere in the colon.[20–22] Numerous biopsies of the region surrounding the area of concern are recommended in evaluating for dysplasia. If these biopsies are positive for dysplasia, local or endoscopic resection is not recommended. A lesion that occurs proximally to known areas of colitis without surrounding inflammation can be considered as sporadic adenoma, and treated endoscopically.

Endoscopically Invisible or Nonresectable Dysplasia

Close involvement of the surgeon, gastroenterologist and pathologist in evaluating dysplasia allows for the best management choices and optimal outcomes. This section focuses on the surgical management of endoscopically invisible or nonresectable dysplasia.

First, it is recommended that a diagnosis of dysplasia (LGD or HGD) be independently confirmed by 2 experienced gastrointestinal pathologists. Controversy continues regarding the management of LGD, owing to the variation in reported rates of progression from LGD to HGD or cancer.[23] Patients confirmed to have endoscopically invisible multifocal LGD or repetitive endoscopically invisible unifocal LGD following evaluation by an expert endoscopist using chromoendoscopy should be counseled and given a strong recommendation for total proctocolectomy.[24] A decision analysis for endoscopically invisible unifocal LGD compared cost-effectiveness of enhanced surveillance with immediate colectomy, and found that immediate colectomy was associated with higher quality-adjusted life years and lower costs.[24] Nonetheless, patients with endoscopically invisible unifocal LGD on surveillance colonoscopy who do not wish to undergo an operation should have the area tattooed, repeat surveillance colonoscopy with chromoendoscopy performed at 3, 6, and 12 months with local and distant biopsies, and then annually.

Before surgical intervention, any patient with a known dysplastic or cancerous lesions should undergo complete colonoscopy surveillance with chromoendoscopy, which allows for best evaluation of where dysplasia may exist. If dysplasia remains endoscopically invisible, a minimum of 3 biopsies every 10 cm is standard; in addition, biopsies of the rectum and anal transition zone should be performed to rule out dysplasia. Multiple biopsies should be performed in any transition zone where an anastomosis may be considered. Surgical options will be based on these findings.

Surgical Options for Resection

Risks of recurrence of disease or findings of synchronous disease must be weighed against the morbidity of surgical resection. Recommendations are generally varied for Crohn's disease and UC, and also vary based on type of dysplasia, morbidities, and patient factors (**Figs. 1** and **2**).

Initial evaluation of patients includes assessment of overall medical stability, fitness for surgery, and current function. Decisions for surgery must be based on the patient's

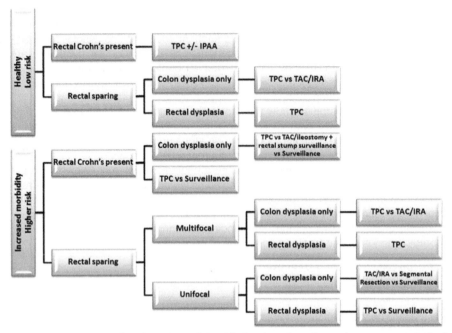

Fig. 1. Surgical options for ulcerative colitis with dysplasia found on colonoscopy. IPAA, ileal pouch anal anastomosis; IRA, ileorectal anastomosis; TAC, total abdominal colectomy; TPC, total proctocolectomy.

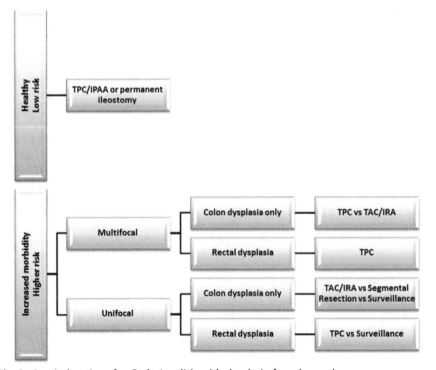

Fig. 2. Surgical options for Crohn's colitis with dysplasia found on colonoscopy.

ability to undergo surgery; in some cases suboptimal procedures will be performed secondary to limited preoperative life expectancy and anticipated comorbidities from undergoing surgery. In addition, assessment of preoperative defecatory dysfunction including incidents of fecal incontinence should be evaluated. Patients with severe preoperative incontinence and difficulty with mobility may benefit most from resection with creation of stomas for functional reasons. Overall goals should be preservation of the quality of life combined with appropriate oncologic resection.

The gold standard for patients from an oncologic perspective is total proctocolectomy with perineal resection and end ileostomy. All colonic mucosa is removed, up to and including mucosa at the anorectal junction, therefore virtually eliminating the risk of colonic metaplasia and advancement to cancer. This result must be weighed against the patient's desire for intestinal continuity. Most patients would prefer to have intestinal continuity, and complete removal of the rectoanal junction would leave them with a permanent colostomy. In addition, though eliminating the risk of concurrent or future colon cancer, in patients with isolated disease or with sporadic adenoma this may not be necessary from an oncologic perspective.

For patients with UC a total proctocolectomy with ileal pouch anal anastomosis is a possibility. This operation removes the colon and colonic mucosa except a small margin at the anorectal junction, and allows for replacement of the rectum with an ileal pouch. The pouch serves as a reservoir to store stool and decrease frequency of defecation for patients. The disadvantages of this procedure include a small risk of recurrence within the rectal mucosa at the margin of the pouch, necessitating regular surveillance; and complication rates of the surgery, which are often 15% or greater and include risk of reoperation, incontinence, decreased fertility, and sexual dysfunction.[25] Some patients with isolated Crohn's colitis and no signs of small intestine or perianal disease may also be appropriate for total proctocolectomy with ileal pouch anal anastomosis These patients are at higher risk of pouch complications such as fistulization, recurrence of pouch inflammation (pouchitis), and pouch failure. To consider this procedure, patients must have good sphincter function at baseline, be surgically fit, and not have signs of low rectal or anal dysplasia on screening biopsies. If HGD is found in the rectum during colonoscopy, reconstruction with ileal pouch anal anastomosis should be delayed to avoid the risk of radiation to the pouch if synchronous advanced carcinoma is found within the rectum after surgical resection. Risks of cancer in the retained rectal mucosa are generally low, reported as less than 5% at 25 years.[26,27] A mucosectomy, or removal of the rectal mucosa down to the anorectal ring, may be performed, but continence may be compromised in this case. In general, patients are expected to have 4 to 6 bowel movements daily, and some soilage or nighttime incontinence is not uncommon.

For patients with diffuse colonic disease but without rectal involvement, it may also be possible to consider a total abdominal colectomy with ileal rectal anastomosis. Advantages of this operation generally include preserved rectal and sexual function. The operation itself is shorter and less extensive. However, this operation does not treat dysplasia or inflammatory disease within the rectum. This area will require continued surveillance, and in patients with both Crohn's disease and UC the rates of recurrence of inflammatory disease in the rectum are as high as 60%.[28] This operation is contraindicated in patients with rectal or anal lesions, and considered as very high risk for patients with multifocal dysplasia. Other contraindications include patients with baseline fecal incontinence or severe rectal inflammation.

For patients who are not fit for anastomosis, or reconnection, a total abdominal colectomy with Hartmann procedure may be performed. This operation leaves the remnant rectum in place during the operation, and an end ileostomy is performed.

Advantages of this surgery include decreased time and morbidity by leaving the rectum in situ. However, risks include inflammation and risk of dysplasia within the rectum, and continued surveillance is necessary.

In isolated inflammatory and dysplastic disease, or in cases of a sporadic adenoma, the most appropriate operation may be a segmental colectomy. Benefits of this operation include shorter operative times, maintenance of key portions of the colon, including possibly the ileocecal valve which may functionally decrease risks of diarrhea, and the greater part of the colon for fluid absorption. This option is restricted to patients with isolated dysplasia and those with relatively normal mucosa in terms of inflammation; surgical anastomosis necessitates functional mucosa for creation of a colon anastomosis. Patients who undergo this option must be committed to continued colonoscopic surveillance to evaluate for metachronous lesions and the risk of continued progression of inflammatory disease. Data demonstrate that up to 40% of patients with Crohn's disease will require additional colectomy at 10 years for recurrence of inflammation after segmental colectomy.[29,30]

All resections, whether segmental or complete proctocolectomies, should follow the principles of surgical oncology. A full lymphadenectomy and vessel resection with high ligation should be completed. Current data recommend resection of a minimum of 12 lymph nodes for segmental colectomy to ensure appropriate staging of tumors.[31]

In addition, good data also exist to affirm that the use of laparoscopic or minimally invasive surgery is beneficial for patients.[32] All of the aforementioned procedures can be performed laparoscopically in experienced hands. Contraindications to laparoscopic surgery are few and decreasing in number, but may include extensive prior adhesions, bulky mesentery, and extraluminal invasion. Benefits of laparoscopy include decreased postoperative pain and quicker return to function; moreover, laparoscopy may allow appropriate patients earlier access to definitive medical oncology treatments.

STRICTURES

The repeated cycle of inflammation, necrosis, and ulceration, alternating with the deposition of granulation tissue during the healing phase, results in the development of raised areas of inflamed tissue that resemble polyps, called pseudopolyps, or may result in stricture formation. Such sequelae make endoscopic surveillance of dysplasia and cancer, and its management, a challenge.

Colonic strictures are more common in Crohn's disease than in UC. Colonic strictures reportedly are found in 5% to 17% of patients with Crohn's colitis.[10] Although data are lacking, colonic strictures have been reported in approximately 5% of UC patients. Rates of stricture occurrence seem to be improving as medical treatments allow more patients to achieve remission. Colonic strictures in any setting should be considered malignant until proven otherwise. Gumaste and colleagues[33] evaluated the Mount Sinai Hospital (New York) population of UC patients with strictures, and found 29% to be malignant. In Crohn's disease, despite a higher rate of stricture occurrence, the rate of malignant colorectal strictures was only 6.8%.[34] There is no role for stricturoplasty in the primary management of colonic strictures in IBD. Strictures found at prior anastomotic sites in Crohn's disease may be judiciously dilated to allow for endoscopic evaluation of recurrence or technical problems from the original resection. Dysplasia and carcinoma at colonic strictures cannot always be detected preoperatively.[35] The stricture must be able to be traversed, adequately examined, and biopsied. Even then, the risk of sampling error in a stricture can be high; a biopsied portion may demonstrate inflammation and fail to show deeper malignancy. If malignancy cannot be excluded, oncologic resection is indicated. In UC, proctocolectomy is the only means to definitively diagnose or rule out carcinoma and to treat possible multifocal malignancy, and should be considered in the management of colonic UC stricture. Unlike UC, a segmental oncologic resection may be appropriate in Crohn's disease colorectal stricture in a patient with limited segmental disease.

SUMMARY

Identification and treatment of dysplasia and colorectal cancer in IBD creates management challenges for the clinician. Treatment options for patients must be based on the understanding of differences in virulence between sporadic adenomas and inflammatory related dysplasia in patients with IBD. Surgical interventions should be based on patient morbidities, location and type of inflammation, and, most importantly, findings of dysplasia. Although the gold standard for oncologic resection is total proctocolectomy, many appropriate options exist that allow for intestinal continuity.

REFERENCES

1. Lennard-Jones JE, Melville DM, Morson BC, et al. Precancer and cancer in extensive ulcerative colitis: findings among 401 patients over 22 years. Gut 1990;31: 800.
2. Odze RD. Diagnostic problems and advances in inflammatory bowel disease. Mod Pathol 2003;16(4):347–58.
3. Ransohoff DF. Colon cancer in ulcerative colitis. Gastroenterology 1988;94: 1089–91.
4. Gyde SN, Prior P, Allan RN, et al. Colorectal cancer in ulcerative colitis: a cohort study of primary referrals from three centers. Gut 1988;29(2):206–17.
5. Jess T, Simonsen J, Jørgensen KT, et al. Decreasing risk of colorectal cancer in patients with inflammatory bowel disease over 30 years. Gastroenterology 2012; 143:375.
6. Choi PM, Zelig MP. Similarity of colorectal cancer in Crohn's disease and ulcerative colitis: implications for carcinogenesis and prevention. Gut 1994;35:950.
7. Greenstein AJ, Sachar DB, Smith H, et al. A comparison of cancer risk in Crohn's disease and ulcerative colitis. Cancer 1981;48:2742.
8. Hamilton SR. Colorectal carcinoma in patients with Crohn's disease. Gastroenterology 1985;89:398.
9. Greenstein AJ. Cancer in inflammatory bowel disease. Mt Sinai J Med 2000; 67(3):227–40.
10. Greenstein AJ. Malignancy in Crohn's disease. Perspect Colon Rectal Surg 1995; 8:137–59.
11. Ekbom A, Helmick C, Zack M, et al. Ulcerative colitis and colorectal cancer. A population-based study. N Engl J Med 1990;323:1228.
12. Ekbom A, Helmick C, Zack M, et al. Increased risk of large-bowel cancer in Crohn's disease with colonic involvement. Lancet 1990;336:357.
13. Bernstein CN, Shanahan F, Weinstein WM. Are we telling patients the truth about surveillance colonoscopy in ulcerative colitis? Lancet 1994;343(8889):71–4.
14. Friedman S, Rubin PH, Bodian C. Screening and surveillance colonoscopy in chronic Crohn's colitis. Gastroenterology 2001;120(4):820–6.
15. Kiran RP, Khoury W, Church JM. Colorectal cancer complicating inflammatory bowel disease: similarities and differences between Crohn's and ulcerative colitis based on three decades of experience. Ann Surg 2010;252(2):330–5.

16. Maykel JA, Hagerman G, Mellgren AF, et al. Crohn's colitis: the incidence of dysplasia and adenocarcinoma in surgical patients. Dis Colon Rectum 2006; 49:950–7.
17. Gorfine SR, Bauer JJ, Harris MT. Dysplasia complicating chronic ulcerative colitis: is immediate colectomy warranted? Dis Colon Rectum 2000;43(11):1575–81.
18. von Herbay A, Herfarth C, Otto HF. Cancer and dysplasia in ulcerative colitis: a histologic study of 301 surgical specimens. Z Gastroenterol 1994;32(7):382–8.
19. Gearhart SL, Nathan H, Pawlik TM, et al. Outcomes from IBD-associated and non-IBD associated colorectal cancer: a Surveillance Epidemiology and End Results Medicare Study. Dis Colon Rectum 2012;55(3):270–7.
20. Engelsgjerd M, Farraye FA, Odze RD. Polypectomy may be adequate treatment for adenoma-like dysplastic lesions in chronic ulcerative colitis. Gastroenterology 1999;117:1288–94.
21. Rubin PH, Friedman S, Harpaz N, et al. Colonoscopic polypectomy in chronic colitis: conservative management after endoscopic resection of dysplastic polyps. Gastroenterology 1999;117:1295.
22. Kitiyakara T, Bailey DM, McIntyre AS, et al. Adenomatous colonic polyps are rare in ulcerative colitis. Aliment Pharmacol Ther 2004;19(8):879–87.
23. Itzkowitz SH, Present DH. Consensus conference: colorectal cancer screening and surveillance in inflammatory bowel disease. Inflamm Bowel Dis 2005;11(3): 314–21.
24. Nguyen GC, Frick KD, Dassopoulos T. Medical decision analysis for the management of unifocal, flat, low-grade dysplasia in ulcerative colitis. Gastrointest Endosc 2009;69:1299.
25. Connelly TM, Koltun WA. The surgical treatment of inflammatory bowel disease-associated dysplasia. Expert Rev Gastroenterol Hepatol 2013;7(4):307–22.
26. Kiesslich R, Neurath MF. Chromoendoscopy in inflammatory bowel disease. Gastroenterol Clin North Am 2012;41(2):291–302.
27. Ziv Y, Fazio VW, Stron SA, et al. Ulcerative colitis and coexisting colorectal cancer: recurrence rate after restorative proctocolectomy. Ann Surg Oncol 1994;1(6):512–5.
28. Pastore RL, Wolff BG, Hodge D. Total abdominal colectomy and ileal rectal anastomosis for inflammatory bowel disease. Dis Colon Rectum 1997;40(12):1455–64.
29. Fichera A, Mccormack R, Rubin MA, et al. Long-term outcome of surgically treated Crohn's colitis: a prospective study. Dis Colon Rectum 2005;4(5):963–9.
30. Prabhakar LP, Laramee C, Nelson H, et al. Avoiding a stoma: role for segmental or abdominal colectomy in Crohn's colitis. Dis Colon Rectum 1997;40(1):71–8.
31. Chang GJ, Rodriguez-Bigas MA, Skibber JM, et al. Lymph node evaluation and survival after curative resection of colon cancer: systematic review. J Natl Cancer Inst 2007;99(6):433–41.
32. Kennedy GD, Heise C, Rajamanickam V, et al. Laparoscopy decreases postoperative complication rates after abdominal colectomy: results from the national surgical quality improvement program. Ann Surg 2009;249(4):596–601.
33. Gumaste V, Sachar DB, Greenstein AJ. Benign and malignant colorectal strictures in ulcerative colitis. Gut 1992;33(7):938–41.
34. Yamazaki Y, Ribeiro MB, Sachar DB, et al. Malignant colorectal strictures in Crohn's disease. Am J Gastroenterol 1991;86(7):882–5.
35. Lashner BA, Turner BC, Bostwick DG, et al. Dysplasia and cancer complicating strictures in ulcerative colitis. Dig Dis Sci 1990;35(3):349–52.

The Unique Pathology of Nonpolypoid Colorectal Neoplasia in IBD

Carlos A. Rubio, MD[a],*, Premysl Slezak, MD[b]

KEYWORDS

- Nonpolypoid colorectal adenomas • IBD • Histopathology • Classification
- Biologic attributes • Experimental studies • Chronologic appearance

KEY POINTS

- Patients with inflammatory bowel disease may develop dysplasia in the cryptal epithelium, polypoid neoplasias, and nonpolypoid (flat) adenomas, lesions at risk to proceed to colorectal carcinoma.
- The onset of invasion in nonpolypoid adenomas may occur without changes in the shape or the size of the lesion.
- In experimental animals, some colonotropic carcinogens induce polypoid and nonpolypoid neoplasias and others induce polypoid neoplasias exclusively.
- Some of the biologic attributes of nonpolypoid adenomas in humans can be demonstrated in laboratory animals.

INTRODUCTION

Patients with inflammatory bowel disease (IBD) (an acronym that includes both ulcerative colitis [UC] and Crohn's colitis [CC]) are at risk to develop dysplasia in the cryptal epithelium, polypoid and nonpolypoid adenomatous growths, and IBD-independent sporadic polypoid and nonpolypoid adenomas. All these lesions may proceed to colorectal carcinoma (CRC).

THE HISTOGENESIS OF CRC IN IBD

Information concerning the histogenesis of CRC in IBD is derived from studies done in patients with UC. At present, 7 alternative pathways have been proposed: (1) from UC-dependent histologically detected dysplastic gland, referred to as dysplasia in flat

[a] Gastrointestinal and Liver Pathology Research Laboratory, Department of Pathology, Karolinska Institute and University Hospital, Stockholm 17176, Sweden; [b] Department of Gastrointestinal Endoscopy, Karolinska University Hospital, Stockholm 17176, Sweden
* Corresponding author. Gastrointestinal and Liver Pathology Research Laboratory, Department of Pathology, Karolinska Institute and University Hospital, Stockholm 17176, Sweden.
E-mail address: Carlos.Rubio@ki.se

Gastrointest Endoscopy Clin N Am 24 (2014) 455–468
http://dx.doi.org/10.1016/j.giec.2014.03.009
giendo.theclinics.com

mucosa in the literature; (2) from UC-dependent adenomatoid neoplastic growths[1]; (3) from UC-independent, age-dependent, sporadic adenomas[1]; (4) from gut-associated lymphoid tissue (GALT)[2]; (5) from nonpolypoid (UC-dependent and UC-independent) adenomas[3]; (6) from UC-dependent discrete villous dysplastic changes[4]; or (7) from apparently nondysplastic mucosa (*de novo* carcinomas).[1]

HISTOLOGICALLY DETECTED DYSPLASIAS IN IBD

Histologically detected dysplasia in IBD may be found in colorectal glands exhibiting parallel tubules or bifurcations; in those instances, the dysplasia is initially found in the basal aspect of the crypts and progresses gradually toward the superficial aspect of the crypts (base-to-surface progression). In mucosa with advanced atrophy without crypts, dysplasia may be found in the superficial epithelium.

A recent search in the literature revealed that most of the publications on flat adenomas in IBD concerned dysplasia in flat mucosa, flat dysplasia, flat dysplastic tissue, or flat low-grade dysplasia. These terms should not be confused with nonpolypoid adenomas, as these adenomas are also flat dysplasias albeit showing a circumscribed clustering of abnormal crypts lined with dysplastic cells. It is crucial to distinguish between these 2 different histologic alterations, as cases of nonpolypoid adenomas are even today being referred to in the literature as flat adenomas. In this article the term "flat" is reserved for nonpolypoid adenomas.

AN EARLY ILLUSTRATION OF NONPOLYPOID ADENOMAS

In 1975, Mr Bussey from the St. Mark's Hospital, London, UK published a monograph on colectomy specimens from patients with familial adenomatous polyposis (FAP). The caption in one of the illustrations reads as follows: "a lesion consisting of adenomatous tubules, which have not produced any thickening of the mucosa". This appears to be the first description of nonpolypoid (flat) colonic adenomas in FAP.[5]

THE PIONEER CLINICAL WORK OF MUTO

In 1985, Muto and colleagues[6] launched the colonoscopic-histologic concept "flat adenoma-carcinoma sequence", uncovering thereby an alternative route to sporadic colorectal carcinogenesis.

THE WESTERN-JAPANESE CONTROVERSY

Hurlstone postulated that the variability in histologic diagnostic criteria used by Western and Japanese pathologists have made comparative studies difficult.[7] To by-pass that difficulty, one of the authors (C.A.R.) sought in 1995, histologic guidance and training on sporadic flat colonic adenomas by Dr Tetsuichiro Muto, Tokyo University, Japan. Subsequently, one of the authors reviewed all sporadic flat adenomas filed at Muto's Department[8] and later examined all sporadic flat adenomas filed at other hospitals in the Tokyo area.[9–11] A total of 1014 flat colorectal lesions were reviewed in Tokyo, which were compared with 600 lesions in Sweden. Those studies revealed that sporadic flat (nonpolypoid) adenomas were more advanced (in terms of high-grade dysplasia [HGD]) and more aggressive (in terms of intramucosal and submucosal invasion) in Japan than in Sweden. Although the causes for the difference in those disparate geographic regions remains debatable, the findings helped us to understand some of the unclear points and discussions that appeared in the literature on this subject.

NONPOLYPOID ADENOMATOUS LESIONS IN IBD DETECTED AT ENDOSCOPY

In 1996, Jaramillo and colleagues[3] detected at endoscopy 104 small polyps in 38 of 85 Swedish patients with UC: 74% were endoscopically flat, 23% polypoid (20% sessile and 3% pedunculated), and in 3% the endoscopic appearance was not recorded. The pathologic examination revealed nonpolypoid (flat) adenomas in 14%, tubular or villous structures with dysplastic cells in the lower part of the crypts in 5%, nonpolypoid hyperplastic polyps in 34%, mucosa with inflammation in 7%, and mucosa in remission in 40%.

SYNCHRONOUS POLYPOID AND NONPOLYPOID ADENOMATOUS LESIONS IN IBD IN COLECTOMY SPECIMENS WITH CARCINOMA

Data show that nonpolypoid adenomatous lesions are commonly found in IBD colectomy specimens with carcinoma. One of the authors has previously reviewed 96 colectomy specimens with UC and carcinoma filed at the Department of Pathology, St Mark's Hospital, London, UK (**Fig. 1**). A total of 3049 sections were available in the 96 colectomy specimens; the mean number of sections/colectomy studied was 31.8 (range 7–97 sections).[1] In addition to carcinomas, several circumscribed adenomatous lesions were found elsewhere in the colon or rectum; they will be referred to as synchronous adenomatous lesions (SALs). Using a low-power examination (4x), the histologic profile of these circumscribed lesions was classified into polypoid and nonpolypoid, both in areas with UC and in areas without inflammation. A total of 104 SALs were found in the 96 colectomies: 73 SALs, which occurred in areas with inflammation, and 31 SALs, in areas without inflammation.

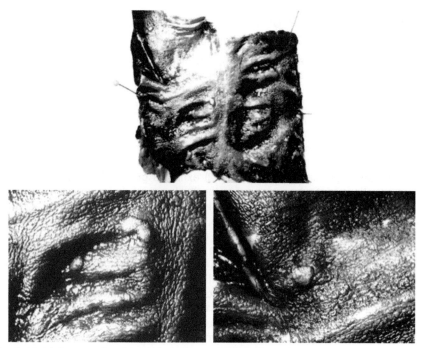

Fig. 1. Multiple nonpolypoid polyps (cecum, after dye spraying, colectomy specimen, natural size).

Polypoid SALs were recorded in 35% (n = 34) of the 96 colectomies. Polypoid SALs in areas with inflammation exhibited irregular dysplastic glands with a jigsaw pattern having irregular bands in the interspersed lamina propria. The mucosa adjacent to these adenomatous lesions showed irregular, dysplastic crypts. Polypoid SALs were found in 47% (n = 34) of the 73 SALs occurring in areas with inflammation.

Polypoid SALs in areas without inflammation had a more regular glandular pattern and the interspersed lamina propria was more regularly distributed, and the adjacent mucosa showed no dysplasia. These polypoid lesions were regarded as sporadic (polypoid) adenomas. Polypoid sporadic adenomas were found in 19% (n = 18) of the 96 colectomies and 58% (n = 18) of the 31 SALs in areas without inflammation.

Nonpolypoid SALs were slightly elevated (en plateau), had discrete villous changes,[4] or were flat-flat. These lesions correspond to type 0 of The Paris endoscopic classification of superficial neoplastic lesions. Nonpolypoid SALs were found in 41% (n = 39) of the 96 colectomies: 53% (n = 39) in the 73 SALs found in areas with inflammation and sporadic adenomas in 42% (n = 13) of the 31 SALs present in areas without inflammation.

Invasive carcinomas were detected in 52% (n = 38) of the 73 SALs found in areas with inflammation and sporadic adenomas in 32% (n = 10) of the 31 SALs recorded in areas without inflammations.[1]

Confirmatory data have been recently collected. In a more recent survey done in Florence, Italy, out of the 39 colectomy specimens with IBD and carcinoma, polypoid SALs were found in 21% (n = 4) of the 19 specimens with UC and in 30% (n = 6) of the 20 colectomies with CC. Nonpolypoid SALs were recorded in 11% (n = 2) of the 19 specimens with UC and in 5% (n = 1) of the 20 colectomies with CC (Rubio, Nesi, in preparation).

HISTOLOGIC CLASSIFICATION OF NONPOLYPOID (FLAT) LESIONS REMOVED AT ENDOSCOPY IN PATIENTS WITHOUT IBD

Because of the relative scarce number of cases of nonpolypoid lesions in IBD reported in the literature, much of the available information on their histologic classification is based on endoscopically removed flat lesions in patients without IBD. The cause of the flat lesions varies greatly. Endoscopically removed flat lesions may disclose nonpolypoid hyperplastic polyps, nonpolypoid serrated polyps, nonpolypoid adenomas (tubular, villous, or serrated), or invasive carcinomas. In this regards, prior observations showed that invasive carcinomas can arise de novo – without surrounding adenomatous tissue.[1]

Nonpolypoid hyperplastic polyps (**Fig. 2**) exhibit a group of tall, straight crypts without serrations, not surpassing twice the thickness of the surrounding mucosa. Nonpolypoid serrated polyps are classified into type 1 (**Fig. 3**), having epithelial serrations in the superficial aspect of the crypts, and type 2, displaying similar glands as those described for sessile serrated polyps (**Fig. 4**). However, because type 2 is usually an intramucosal lesion, the term sessile serrated polyp cannot be applied.

Nonpolypoid adenomas (**Fig. 5**) denote a circumscribed cluster of abnormal crypts lined with dysplastic cells having proliferative, biochemical, and molecular aberrations; they are surrounded by nondysplastic mucosa. In well-oriented sections, nonpolypoid adenomas may appear slightly elevated, with a height not surpassing twice the thickness of the nondysplastic surrounded mucosa, or depressed. Based on the structural configuration of the crypts, these adenomas are classified into tubular, villous, or serrated. Paneth cell adenoma and fenestrated adenoma are 2 unusual phenotypes of nonpolypoid adenomas.[8,12]

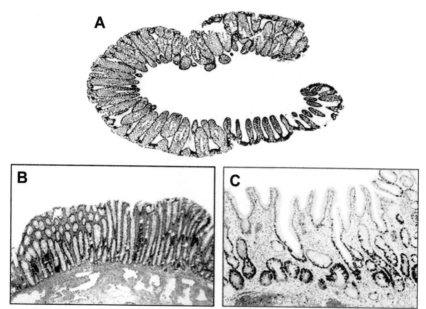

Fig. 2. (*A–C*) Nonpolypoid hyperplastic polyps, with straight crypts, without serrations. The crypts are somewhat wider at the luminal aspect than at the base of the polyp, (*C*) immunostain showing cell proliferation at the base of the hyperplastic crypts (colon, mucosectomies, Ki 67 immunostain, batch MIB1, original magnification ×10) ([*A*] Hematoxylin and eosin, original magnification ×2; [*B*] hematoxylin and eosin, original magnification ×4).

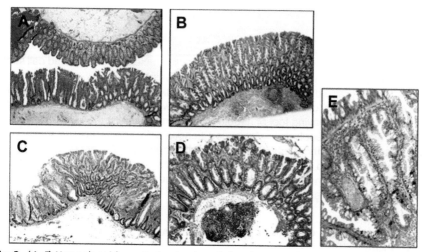

Fig. 3. (*A–E*) Nonpolypoid serrated polyp type 1 showing serrations in the upper part of the crypts. Note absence of cellular dysplasia (colon). (*A*) Nonpolypoid serrated polyp type 1 (lower part); compare with the normal colonic mucosa (upper part, colectomy specimen) ([*A*] Hematoxylin and eosin, original magnification ×2; [*B–D*] Hematoxylin and eosin, original magnification ×4; [*E*] Hematoxylin and eosin, original magnification ×10).

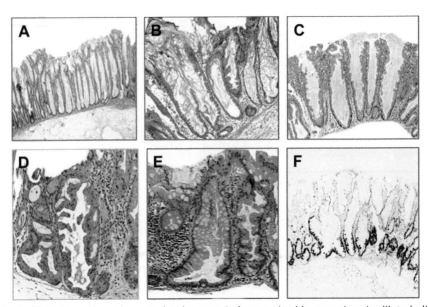

Fig. 4. (*A–D*) Nonpolypoid serrated polyp type 2 characterized by serrations in dilated, distorted crypts replenished by mucus. The basal aspect of the crypts is wider than the luminal aspect. Serrations may reach the lower portion of the crypts. Note absence of cellular dysplasia. The covering luminal mucus may conceal the polyp at endoscopic examination. Nonpolypoid serrated polyp type 2 has the histologic characteristics of sessile serrated polyps. However, as it only occupies the normal thickness of the colonic mucosa, nonpolypoid serrated polyp type 2 is an intramucosal, nonsessile lesion, (*E*) base of a crypt with horizontal (lateral) bifurcation, (*F*) immunostain showing cell proliferation at the base of the crypts (colon, nonpolypoid serrated polyp type 2, Ki 67 immunostain, batch MIB1) ([*A*] Hematoxylin and eosin, original magnification ×2; [*B,C,F*] Hematoxylin and eosin, original magnification ×4; [*D,E*] Hematoxylin and eosin, original magnification ×10).

DYSPLASIA AND CARCINOMA IN COLORECTAL NONPOLYPLOID ADENOMAS

On the basis of the degree of severity of intraepithelial nuclear aberration and cell stratification, dysplasia in nonpolypoid adenomas is classified into low-grade dysplasia (LGD) and high-grade dysplasia (HGD). The dysplastic cells in HGD may exhibit either hyperchromatic nuclei or hypochromatic nuclei showing a large nucleolus. Colorectal adenomas with HGD having foci of neoplastic cells in the *lamina propria mucosae* are called intramucosal neoplasia.[13] Advanced nonpolypoid adenomas are those adenomas having HGD without or with intramucosal neoplasia.[14] Advanced nonpolypoid adenomas are prone to evolve into invasive carcinoma. Invasive carcinomas are those showing tumor cells and /or glands penetrating through the *muscularis mucosa*, and invading the submucosal tissues or beyond.

BIOLOGIC ATTRIBUTES OF NONPOLYPOID ADENOMAS
Acidic Mucins

One important function of the colorectal mucosa is to produce acidic mucins. Sections from flat adenomas were stained with alcian blue pH 2.5 (AB) to highlight sialomucins and with high iron diamine to evidence sulfomucins. Acid mucins were found in the upper and lower parts of the crypts in all sections having normal colonic mucosa, flat

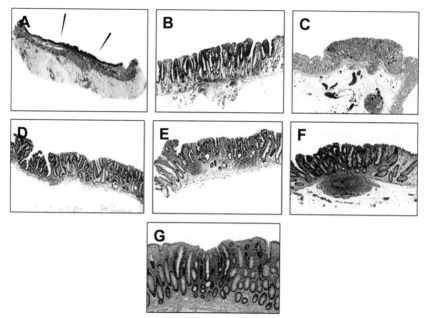

Fig. 5. (*A–G*) Nonpolypoid tubular adenomas exhibiting various degrees of cellular dysplasia (colon). *A*, arrows limit the area with nonpolypoid adenoma ([*A*] Hematoxylin and eosin, colectomy specimen, natural size; [*B–F*] Hematoxylin and eosin, original magnification ×4; [*G*] Hematoxylin and eosin, original magnification ×10).

hyperplastic polyps, and flat serrated polyps. Acid mucins were also found in the upper part of the crypts in 72% of the flat serrated adenomas, but in none of the flat tubular adenomas. In contrast, acid mucins were found in the lower part of the crypts in 90% of flat tubular adenomas, but in none of the flat serrated adenomas. These findings indicate that acidic mucin production is partially depleted in flat adenomas and that the depletion in flat tubular adenomas differs topographically from that in flat serrated adenomas.[15]

Cell Proliferation

All colorectal adenomas display increased cell proliferation. When sections from flat adenomas were challenged with Ki 67 (batch MIB1) (**Fig. 6**), high cell proliferation was found in the upper part of the crypts of flat tubular adenomas and in the lower part in flat serrated adenomas with or without invasive carcinoma.[16] Because of these findings it was conceived that the dysplastic cells of the lower portion of the serrated crypts might be genuine neoplastic cells, prone to invade the host.

p53

Mutation of the p53 gene in adenomas is associated with late progression to carcinoma. When flat adenomas were challenged with the protein encoded by the *TP53* gene, 62% of the flat tubular adenomas with HGD, 67% of the flat (traditional) serrated adenomas with HGD, and all carcinomas arising in those adenomas overexpressed p53. Thus, a high proportion of flat adenomas (tubular and serrated) and resulting carcinomas concur (**Figs. 7–10**) with mutation of the p53 protein.[17]

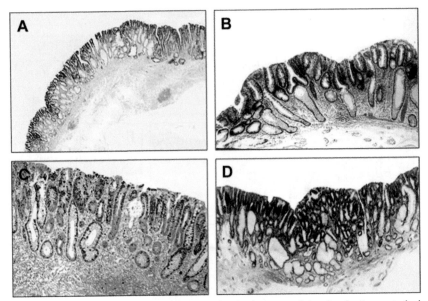

Fig. 6. (A–D) Cell proliferation starting at the luminal aspect of the dysplastic crypts (colon, nonpolypoid tubular adenomas, Ki 67 immunostain, batch MIB1).

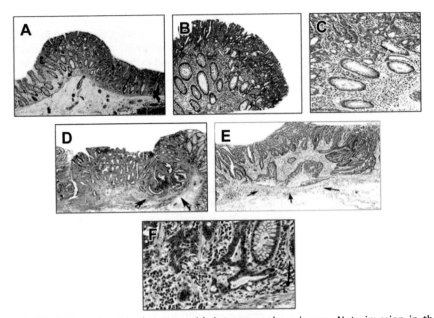

Fig. 7. (A–C) Nonpolypoid adenomas with intramucosal carcinoma. Note invasion in the *lamina propria* without invasion of the submucosal layer. (D–F) show no invasion or penetration of the *muscularis mucosa* (at *arrows*) ([A,D,E] Hematoxylin and eosin, original magnification ×2; [B] Hematoxylin and eosin, original magnification ×4; [C] Hematoxylin and eosin, original magnification ×10).

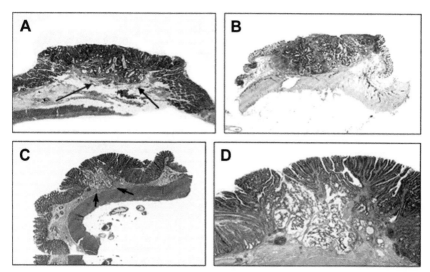

Fig. 8. (*A–D*) Nonpolypoid adenomas, with invasive carcinoma in the submucosal layer. Arrows show invasive carcinoma in *A* and *C*. ([*A–C*] Hematoxylin and eosin, original magnification ×2; [*D*] Hematoxylin and eosin, original magnification ×10).

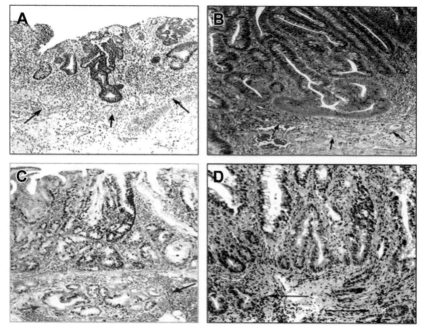

Fig. 9. (*A–D*) Nonpolypoid neoplasias in UC. (*A, B*) Intramucosal invasion. Note lack of invasion of the *muscularis mucosa*, (*B–D*) neoplastic glands invading the submucosal layer (at *arrows*) ([*A,D*] Hematoxylin and eosin, original magnification ×4; [*B*] Hematoxylin and eosin, original magnification ×10; [*C*] Ki67 immunostain, original maginification ×2).

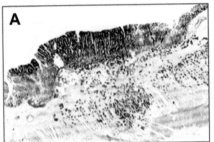
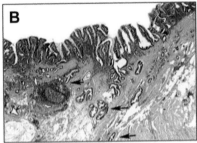
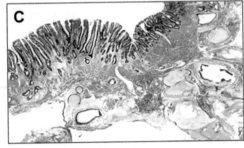

Fig. 10. (*A–C*) Nonpolypoid adenoma with carcinoma invading the *muscularis propria* (UC, MNF 116, immunostain, original magnification ×2); (*B*) nonpolypoid villous dysplasia with invasive carcinoma at *arrows* (UC); and (*C*) nonpolypoid villous dysplasia with mucus-producing adenocarcinoma (UC) ([*B*] Hematoxylin and eosin, original magnification ×2; [*C*] Hematoxylin and eosin, original magnification ×4).

Collagenesis and Microangiogenesis

In the mesenchymal core of polypoid adenomas, both collagen (the principal and most abundant component of the connective tissue) and microvessels are markedly increased. In contrast, none to slightly increased collagen and microvessels are found in nonpolypoid adenomas. Because molecular signals released from mesenchymal cells evoke collagenesis and those from neoplastic cells, microangiogenesis, it was entertained that 2 disparate molecular signals are instrumental in triggering collagenesis and microangiogenesis in the mesenchymal core of polypoid adenomas. The paucity of collagenesis and microangiogenesis in nonpolypoid adenomas suggest that these 2 molecular signals are either inadequately or not elaborated, elaborated but not released, or locally abrogated.[18]

Lymphocytic Infiltration

Intraepithelial lymphocytes (IELs) are often seen in polypoid and nonpolypoid adenomas. Nonpolypoid adenomas with HGD contain more IELs than those with LGD, implying that the degree of IEL infiltration increases with increasing degree of dysplastic severity and/or with the increasing biologic age of the adenoma. Notably, 38% of the nonpolypoid adenomas exhibited a subjacent lymphoid aggregate.[19] It is not inconceivable that lymphoid aggregates might evolve as an immunologic mucosal response, as do occur in newly formed lymphoid aggregates in CC.[20]

Apoptosis

Intraepithelial granules (Leuchtenberger bodies) are often found in polypoid and nonpolypoid adenomas. In a survey, 84% of the nonpolypoid (flat) adenomas exhibited apoptotic granules. The overwhelming majority of the apoptotic granules were seen in the subnuclear basal aspect of the dysplastic cells facing the basement membrane, denoting that the cells responsible for the apoptotic granules were to be found in the vicinity of the lamina propria normally infiltrated by lymphocytes.[21] Direct immunoperoxidase detection of nuclear DNA fragmentation and transmission electron microscopy comfirmed that these DNA-containing bodies were apoptotic (nuclear) fragments from disintegrated lymphocytes, and not nuclear remnants from dead dysplastic cells.[22] In fact, dysplastic cells remained undamaged (as deduced from transmission electronmicroscopy and nuclear DNA proliferation markers).

Semiquantitative assessments of apoptotic granules showed that the number of flat adenomas with excessive granular density was highest amongst those with HGD. Hence, apoptosis in nonpolypoid adenomas might express a mechanism of cell defense, whereby neoplastic cells inflict apoptosis on IEL in advanced nonpolypoid adenomas, through the Fas-FasL pathway.[23]

Importantly, the frequency of apoptotic granules in flat adenomas is similar in Japan and Sweden, implying that apoptosis in those lesions neither is influenced by race nor by the environment.

K-RAS

The authors demonstrated a low K-*ras* mutation rate in flat adenomas. Cancers arising *de novo* were significantly associated with loss of heterozygosity at chromosome 3p.[24]

LESSONS FROM THE ANIMAL WORLD

The chronologic appearance of flat adenomas was traced in a cohort of rats injected with dimethylhydrazine (DMH). Flat adenomas developed earlier (week 13) than polypoid adenomas (week 15). Flat adenomas were more numerous on week 19, whereas polypoid adenomas were more numerous on week 22.[25]

Polypoid carcinomas evolved earlier (week 15) than flat carcinomas (week 19), and on week 22, 63% of the carcinomas were polypoid but only 25% were flat carcinomas.

Flat adenomas in right colon progressed more rapidly to invasive carcinoma than polypoid adenomas, whereas protruding adenomas in the left colon progressed more rapidly to invasive carcinoma than flat adenomas.[25]

BIOLOGIC ATTRIBUTES OF NONPROTRUDING ADENOMAS IN RATS
Lymphocytic Infiltration and Apoptosis

IELs and apoptotic granules were found in 95% and 98% of the tumors induced by GLU, a mutagen of glutamic acid, but only in 21% of DMH-induced neoplasias. The presence of IELs and apoptotic granules in GLU-induced tumors, and their absence in most of the DMH tumors, is puzzling. However, GLU neoplasias were induced by daily doses for 24 months, whereas DMH neoplasias by weekly doses, for up to 6 months. It would appear that "slowly growing" colonic GLU neoplasias often attract IELs leading to apoptosis, whereas "rapidly growing" DMH tumors seldom elicit those reactions.[26,27]

Acid Mucins

AB-stained sections from the colon of rats with simultaneously growing tumors were quantified in an image analyzer. The AB-positive areas occupied only 35% of the mucosa, both in tumor-bearing rats and in nontumor-bearing DMH-treated rats, suggesting that the decrease of mucin production might be related either to the protracted DMH treatment or to a genuine biochemical premalignant change in the colonic mucosa.[28]

Colonotropic Carcinogens and Flat Adenomas

After DMH injection to 278 rats, 358 neoplasias developed. Of the 60 colonic adenomas, 25% were flat adenomas, and of the 298 colonic carcinomas, 13% were flat carcinomas originating in flat adenomas, 28% protruding carcinomas, and the remaining 30% lymphoid-associated carcinomas (originating in GALT).

After GLU treatment to 112 rats, 52 polypoid adenomas and 11 polypoid carcinomas evolved; flat neoplasias did not develop.[27] Taken together, these animal studies suggest that DMH might be the carcinogen of choice to recreate the human model of carcinogenesis, namely nonpolypoid neoplasias, polypoid neoplasias, and GALT carcinomas. The limitation is that DMH elicits in rats a high percentage of GALT carcinomas, a phenotype that infrequently occurs in the human counterpart.[29]

Of particular interest is the recent finding of Iishi and colleagues[30] in rats; using azoxymethane and pravastatin, an inhibitor of ras p21 isoprenylation, an increased number of flat adenomas was achieved.

SUMMARY

Because few cases of nonpolypoid adenomas are being detected and followed in IBD, it remains unknown whether these adenomas develop before, simultaneously, or after the appearance of histologically detected dysplasias or adenomatoid neoplasias. The design of new animal models might be of help in obtaining this basic information.

ACKNOWLEDGMENTS

To Drs Tetsuichiro Muto, Teruyuki Hirota, Yo Kato, Tomo Kitagawa, Kyoichi Nakamura, Haruo Sugano, Shozo Takayama, and Takatoshi Ishikawa, Tokyo, Japan. Their guidance, co-operation, and generosity have permitted to compile this article.

REFERENCES

1. Rubio CA. Serrated neoplasias and de novo carcinomas in ulcerative colitis: a histological study in colectomy specimens. J Gastroenterol Hepatol 2007;22(7): 1024–31.
2. Rubio CA, Befrits R, Ericsson J. Carcinoma in gut-associated lymphoid tissue in ulcerative colitis: Case report and review of literature. World J Gastrointest Endosc 2013;5:293–6.
3. Jaramillo E, Watanabe M, Befrits R, et al. Small, flat colorectal neoplasias in long-standing ulcerative colitis detected by high-resolution electronic video endoscopy. Gastrointest Endosc 1996;44(1):15–22.
4. Hamamoto N, Rubio CA, Befrits R, et al. Subtle villous changes detected at endoscopy in patients with inflammatory bowel disease. Dig Endosc 2005; 17(Suppl 1):34–9.
5. Bussey HJ. Familial polyposis colon. Baltimore (MD): Johns Hopkins University Press; 1975.
6. Muto T, Kamiya J, Sawada T, et al. Small "flat adenoma" of the large bowel with special reference to its clinicopathologic features. Dis Colon Rectum 1985; 28(11):847–51.

7. Hurlstone DP. The detection of flat and depressed colorectal lesions: which endoscopic imaging approach? Gastroenterology 2008;135(2):338–43.

8. Rubio CA, Kato Y, Hirota T, et al. Histologic classification of endoscopically removed flat colorectal polyps: a multicentric study. Jpn J Cancer Res 1996; 87(8):849–55.

9. Rubio CA, Kumagai J, Kanamori T, et al. Flat adenomas and flat adenocarcinomas of the colorectal mucosa in Japanese and Swedish patients. Comparative histologic study. Dis Colon Rectum 1995;38(10):1075–9.

10. Rubio CA, Kato Y, Hirota T, et al. Flat serrated adenomas of the colorectal mucosa in Japanese patients. In Vivo 1996;10(3):339–43.

11. Rubio CA, Saito Y, Watanabe M, et al. Non-polypoid colorectal neoplasias: a multicentric study. Anticancer Res 1999;19(3B):2361–4.

12. Rubio CA, Kanter L, Björk J, et al. Paneth cell-rich flat adenoma of the rectum: report of a case. Jpn J Cancer Res 1996;87(1):109–12.

13. Rubio CA, Nesi G, Messerini L, et al. The Vienna classification applied to colorectal adenomas. J Gastroenterol Hepatol 2006;21(11):1697–703.

14. Rubio CA, Kristjansdottir S, Thodleifsson B, et al. The frequency of advanced adenoma in consulting patients: a nationwide survey in Iceland (2003-2006). Colorectal Dis 2012;14(9):e595–602.

15. Rubio CA, Slezak P, Rodensjö M. Differences in the distribution of acidic mucins between flat tubular adenomas and flat serrated adenomas of the colorectal mucosa. In Vivo 1996;10(3):383–8.

16. Rubio CA, Rodensjö M. Flat serrated adenomas and flat tubular adenomas of the colorectal mucosa: differences in the pattern of cell proliferation. Jpn J Cancer Res 1995;86(8):756–60.

17. Rubio CA, Rodensjö M. Mutation of p53 tumor suppressor gene in flat neoplastic lesions of the colorectal mucosa. Dis Colon Rectum 1996;39(2):143–7.

18. Rubio CA. Differences in angiogenesis and collagenesis between exophytic and flat adenomas of the colorectal mucosa. Anticancer Res 1997;17(1B):737–42.

19. Rubio CA, Kato Y, Hirota T. Intraepithelial lymphocytes in flat colorectal adenomas. In Vivo 1997;11(5):393–4.

20. Rubio CA, Ásmundsson J, Silva P, et al. Lymphoid aggregates in Crohn's colitis and mucosal immunity. Virchows Arch 2013;463(5):637–42.

21. Rubio CA, Kumagai J, Nakamura K, et al. Leuchtenberger bodies in flat adenomas of the colorectal mucosa: a comparison between Japanese and Swedish patients. Jpn J Cancer Res 1996;87(6):618–22.

22. Rubio CA. Intraepithelial lymphocytes vs. colorectal neoplastic cells: who is winning the apoptotic battle? Apoptosis 1997;2(6):489–93.

23. Rubio CA. Tumor cells induce apoptosis in lymphocytes. Nat Med 1997;3(3): 253–4.

24. Yashiro M, Carethers JM, Laghi L, et al. Genetic pathways in the evolution of morphologically distinct colorectal neoplasms. Cancer Res 2001;61(6):2676–83.

25. Shetye J, Rubio CA. The chronological appearance of flat colonic neoplasias in rats. In Vivo 2004;18(2):197–202.

26. Rubio CA. Apoptotic differences in experimentally induced colorectal rat tumours. Apoptosis 1998;3(1):35–9.

27. Rubio CA, Takayama S. Difference in histology and size in colonic tumors of rats receiving two different carcinogens. J Environ Pathol Toxicol Oncol 1994;13(3): 191–7.

28. Rubio CA, Rivera F. Quantification of acid mucins in the descending colon of rats having simultaneously growing colonic tumors. APMIS 1991;99(11):993–6.

29. Rubio CA, Lindh C, Björk J, et al. Protruding and non-protruding colon carcinomas originating in gut-associated lymphoid tissue. Anticancer Res 2010; 30(7):3019–22.

30. Iishi H, Tatsuta M, Baba M, et al. ras p21 Isoprenylation inhibition induces flat colon tumors in Wistar rats. Dis Colon Rectum 2000;43(1):70–5.

Toward a Consensus on Endoscopic Surveillance of Patients with Colonic Inflammatory Bowel Disease

Amandeep K. Shergill, MD, MS[a],*, Francis A. Farraye, MD, MSc[b]

KEYWORDS

- IBD-associated colorectal neoplasia ● IBD-associated colorectal cancer
- Colitis surveillance ● Colonoscopy ● Chromoendoscopy

KEY POINTS

- All patients with ulcerative colitis (UC) and Crohn's colitis should be offered a screening colonoscopy 8 to 10 years after onset of disease symptoms to restage extent of disease and evaluate for endoscopic features that confer an increased risk for inflammatory bowel disease–associated colorectal neoplasia (IBD-CRN).
- Surveillance colonoscopy should be offered to UC patients with left-sided or extensive colitis (thus excluding patients with isolated proctitis), and for patients with Crohn's colitis involving more than 1 segment of the colon or at least one-third of the colon.
- Patients with the highest risk of IBD-CRN should undergo annual surveillance. Lower-risk patients can undergo surveillance at less frequent intervals, every 2 to 5 years.
- European and Australian guidelines agree that dye-based chromoendoscopy with targeted biopsies maximizes detection of colorectal neoplasia during surveillance colonoscopy, and is the surveillance method of choice. Most United States guidelines endorse chromoendoscopy with targeted biopsy as an option for surveillance.
- Endoscopically visible lesions that are well circumscribed and amenable to endoscopic resection with no evidence of dysplasia in the surrounding flat mucosa or elsewhere in the colon are appropriate for continued colonoscopic surveillance.

INTRODUCTION

Endoscopic surveillance for colitis-associated colorectal neoplasia (CRN) and colorectal cancer (CRC) is recommended by multiple national and international

[a] Department of Medicine, University of California, San Francisco, San Francisco VA Medical Center, 4150 Clement Street (VA 111B), San Francisco, CA 94121, USA; [b] Department of Medicine, Boston University School of Medicine, Section of Gastroenterology Boston Medical Center, 85 East Concord Street, 7th Floor Boston, MA 02118, USA
* Corresponding author.
E-mail address: amandeep.shergill@ucsf.edu

Gastrointest Endoscopy Clin N Am 24 (2014) 469–481
http://dx.doi.org/10.1016/j.giec.2014.03.006
1052-5157/14/$ – see front matter Published by Elsevier Inc.

gastrointestinal (GI) societies.[1–8] The goal of endoscopic surveillance is to reduce the morbidity and mortality of CRC, by either detecting and resecting dysplasia or detecting CRC at earlier, potentially curable stages.[9] Randomized controlled trials (RCTs) assessing the efficacy of surveillance colonoscopy in IBD have not been performed, and likely will not be performed.[6] Case series, case-control studies, and population-based cohort studies suggest that use of surveillance colonoscopy is associated with an earlier stage of cancer diagnosis and improved CRC-related survival in IBD patients.[10–14] Although a Cochrane analysis from 2006 concluded that there is no clear evidence that surveillance colonoscopy prolongs survival in patients with extensive colitis,[15] a subsequent cohort study of 149 patients with IBD-associated CRC from the Netherlands, not included in the Cochrane analysis, found a 100% 5-year survival of 23 patients enrolled in a surveillance program before CRC detection, compared with 74% in a nonsurveillance group ($P = .042$).[14] Of 30 CRC-related deaths during the study period (January 1, 1990 to July 1, 2006), only 1 patient was in the surveillance group compared with 29 in the nonsurveillance group ($P = .047$). It was also noted that 52% of patients in the surveillance group had Stage 0 to 1 CRC, compared with 24% in the nonsurveillance group ($P = .004$).[14] In an exploratory cost-effectiveness model performed by the National Institute for Health and Clinical Excellence (NICE), colonoscopy surveillance was determined to be cost-effective for high-risk groups, which included IBD patients with any history of dysplasia, extensive active colitis, primary sclerosing cholangitis (PSC), strictures within the last 5 years, or family history of CRC before 50 years of age.[6]

Thus, surveillance colonoscopy in patients with ulcerative colitis (UC) and Crohn's colitis has been recommended by multiple societies in the United States (American Gastroenterological Society [AGA],[2] American Society for Gastrointestinal Endoscopy multiple European societies (British Society for Gastroenterology [BSG],[1] NICE,[6] European Crohn's and Colitis Organization [ECCO][7]), the [ASGE],[5] American College of Gastroenterology [ACG],[4] Crohn's and Colitis Foundation of America [CCFA],[3] multiple European societies [British Society for Gastroenterology (BSG),[1] NICE,[6] European Crohn's and Colitis Organization (ECCO)],[7] the Cancer Council of Australia [CCA],[8] the New Zealand Guidelines Group,[16] and the North American Society for Pediatric Gastroenterology, Hepatology and Nutrition [NASPGHN]).[17] However, recommendations differ in regards to timing of initial screening colonoscopy, recommended surveillance intervals, optimal technique for dysplasia detection, and management of detected lesions and endoscopically invisible dysplasia. This article reviews current society guidelines, highlighting similarities and differences, in an attempt to form a general consensus on surveillance for patients with IBD, while drawing attention to controversial areas in need of further research.

WHO SHOULD BE OFFERED SCREENING AND SURVEILLANCE FOR IBD-ASSOCIATED CRC?

Most societies agree that all patients with a history of UC (even isolated proctitis) and Crohn's colitis should be offered a screening colonoscopy approximately 8 to 10 years after the onset of clinical symptoms to re-stage extent of disease and evaluate for endoscopic features that confer a higher risk for IBD-associated CRN (IBD-CRN). The exception is the NICE guideline,[6] which recommends only offering colonoscopic surveillance to patients with Crohn's colitis involving more than 1 segment of the colon or left-sided or more extensive UC, but not isolated ulcerative proctitis. All societies recommend that patients with PSC and UC should be enrolled in a surveillance program at the time of diagnosis.

During the initial screening examination, restaging biopsies are recommended to determine disease extent and severity. The extent of disease is defined by the maximum documented extent of disease on any colonoscopy. All societies recommend surveillance colonoscopy for UC patients with left-sided or extensive colitis (thus excluding patients with isolated proctitis),[1–6,8] and for Crohn's colitis involving more than 1 segment of the colon[6,18] or at least one-third of the colon.[2,3,5,8] The BSG considers patients with Crohn's disease of less than 50% of colonic involvement, regardless of grade of inflammation, as lower risk, but does offer surveillance at the longest (5-year) intervals.[1] The ACG guidelines recognize the possible increased risk of cancer in long-standing Crohn's disease, but state that surveillance guidelines have yet to be defined, and do not endorse a screening or surveillance strategy.[19]

Guidelines Summary

- All patients with UC and Crohn's colitis should be offered a screening colonoscopy to restage the extent of disease and evaluate for endoscopic features that confer a higher risk for IBD-CRN.
- Surveillance colonoscopy should be offered for UC patients with left-sided or extensive colitis (thus excluding patients with isolated proctitis), and for Crohn's colitis involving more than 1 segment of the colon or at least one-third of the colon.

WHEN SHOULD SCREENING BE INITIATED?

Current guidelines base screening for IBD-CRN primarily on duration of disease. The risk of IBD-CRN increases over time, although estimates of risk vary in the literature. Meta-analysis of older studies estimated an increase in risk over time, with a cumulative CRC risk of 2% at 10 years, 8% at 20 years, and 18% after 30 years of colitis.[20] More recent population-based studies have demonstrated a lower overall risk, from 2.5% at 20 years, to 7.6% at 30 years, and 10.8% at 40 years of extensive UC.[21]

These studies support initiating screening by 10 years of symptom onset, as recommended by the BSG[1] and NICE,[6] with most societies recommending initiating screening at 8 years[2,8,18] or 8 to 10 years[3–5] after symptom onset. However, recent population-based studies demonstrating that 17% to 35%[22–24] of patients develop CRC before 8 to 10 years has prompted some societies to recommend earlier screening colonoscopy. The NASPGHN recommends initiation of screening 7 to 10 years after diagnosis.[17] The 2012 Second European evidence-based consensus on the diagnosis and management of UC states that screening could be initiated 6 to 8 years after symptom onset, taking into consideration risk factors such as extent and severity of disease, history of pseudopolyps, family history, and age at onset.[7]

These recent studies demonstrating early IBD-CRN occurrence underscore the need for considering additional risk factors to optimize initiation of IBD-CRN screening. Risk stratification based on age at disease onset (both young age and older age appear to confer increased risk[23,25]), extent and severity of disease, family history, and pseudopolyps has been advocated by some of the societies, and is in need of further study for incorporation into the IBD surveillance guidelines.

Guidelines Summary

- Most society guidelines recommend initiating surveillance 8 to 10 years after disease onset; some recommend considering risk factors that may increase the risk for IBD-CRN, and warrant earlier surveillance.

HOW OFTEN SHOULD SURVEILLANCE COLONOSCOPY BE PERFORMED?

Optimal surveillance intervals have not been defined in prospective studies, and the societies differ on their recommended surveillance intervals after the index screening colonoscopy. In general, patients with the highest risk of IBD-CRN are recommended for annual surveillance, whereas patients with the lowest risk are recommended for less frequent surveillance intervals, varying from 2 to 5 years.

Risk factors for IBD-CRN include concomitant PSC, extensive colitis, active endoscopic or histologic inflammation, a family history of CRC in a first-degree relative before 50 years of age, personal history of dysplasia, presence of strictures on colonoscopy, and, possibly, gender (**Table 1**). With the exception of gender, all recent guidelines recommend annual surveillance for individuals with these high risk features (AGA, BSG, NICE, ECCO, CCA).

Normal-appearing mucosa on surveillance appears to be associated with a decreased risk of IBD-CRN, reduced to approximately that of the general population.[34] The United States GI societies have not yet endorsed lengthening surveillance intervals beyond 3 years. BSG, ECCO, NICE and CCA recommend a risk-stratified approach to cancer surveillance, and increase the surveillance interval to 5 years in the lowest-risk patients (**Table 2**).

Severe active inflammation, prior dysplasia, and strictures are universally accepted as high-risk endoscopic features. Whereas the CCA[8] suggests annual examinations for patients with multiple pseudopolyps and shortened colons, the BSG[1] and the ECCO[18] guidelines consider these patients for colonoscopies every 2 to 3 years. The CCA[8] allows for a 5-year interval for surveillance in patients with 2 prior macroscopically and histologically normal colonoscopies, whereas the NICE[6] and BSG[1] consider patients with left-sided UC or Crohn's disease of similar extent, regardless of degree of inflammation, appropriate for 5-year surveillance.

Table 1
Risk factors for IBD-CRN

Risk Factor	Risk of IBD-CRN	Authors,[Ref.] Year
PSC	OR 4.09, 95% CI 2.89–5.67	Soetikno et al,[26] 2002
Extensive colitis	Pancolitis associated with a SIR 5.6–14.8 compared with the general population	Ekbom et al,[27] 1990 Soderlund et al,[28] 2009 Beaugerie et al,[24] 2013
Active endoscopic inflammation	OR 2.54, 95% CI 1.45–4.44	Rutter et al,[29] 2004
Active histologic inflammation	OR 5.13, 95% CI 2.36–11.14 OR 2.56, 95% CI 1.45–4.54 HR 3.0, 95% CI 1.4–6.3 for mean inflammatory score	Rutter et al,[29] 2004 Rubin et al,[30] 2013 Gupta et al,[31] 2007
Family history of CRC <50 y old	RR 9.2, 95% CI 3.7–23	Askling et al,[32] 2001
Personal history of dysplasia	LGD: 12-fold increased risk of developing advanced neoplasia and 9-fold increased risk of developing CRC	Thomas et al,[33] 2007
Strictures on colonoscopy	OR 4.62, 95% CI 1.03–20.8	Rutter et al,[34] 2004
Gender	Men: SIR 2.6, 95% CI 2.2–3.0 Women: SIR 1.9, 95% CI 1.5–2.3	Jess et al,[25] 2012

Abbreviations: CI, confidence interval; CRC, colorectal cancer; HR, hazard ratio; IBD-CRN, inflammatory bowel disease–associated colorectal neoplasia; LGD, low-grade dysplasia; OR, odds ratio; PSC, primary sclerosing cholangitis; RR, relative risk; SIR, standardized incidence ratio.

Table 2
Risk-stratified approach to IBD-CRN surveillance

	Every Year: High Risk	Every 3 Years: Intermediate Risk	Every 5 Years: Low Risk
BSG,[1] 2010	Moderate or severe endoscopic/histologic active inflammation Stricture within the past 5 y Confirmed dysplasia within the past 5 y in a patient who declines surgery PSC Family history of CRC in first-degree relative <50 y	Mild endoscopic/histologic inflammation Presence of postinflammatory polyps Family history of CRC in first-degree relative >50 y	No endoscopic/histologic active inflammation (histologic chronic or quiescent changes acceptable) Left-sided colitis (any grade of inflammation) Crohn's colitis affecting <50% surface area of the colon (any grade of inflammation)
NICE,[6] 2011	Extensive ulcerative or Crohn's colitis with moderate or severe active inflammation PSC Colonic strictures in the past 5 y Any grade of dysplasia in the past 5 y CRC in first-degree relative <50 y	Extensive ulcerative or Crohn's colitis with mild active inflammation Postinflammatory polyps CRC in first-degree relative >50 y	Left-sided UC or Crohn's colitis of similar extent Extensive but quiescent UC/Crohn's colitis
ECCO,[18] 2013	Stricture or dysplasia detected within past 5 y PSC Extensive colitis with severe active inflammation CRC in first-degree relative <50 y	Every 2–3 y recommended Extensive colitis with mild or moderate active inflammation Postinflammatory polyps CRC in first-degree relative >50 y	Neither intermediate- nor high-risk features
CCA,[8] 2011	Active disease PSC CRC in first-degree relative <50 y Colonic stricture Multiple postinflammatory polyps or shortened colon (endoscopic features of prior severe inflammation) Previous dysplasia	Inactive UC or Crohn's colitis affecting more than one-third of the colon without any high-risk features CRC in first-degree relative >50 y	Two prior colonoscopies that were macroscopically and histologically normal

A minimum of 1 factor is needed to meet criteria defined as high, intermediate, or low risk.
Abbreviations: BSG, British Society for Gastroenterology; CCA, Cancer Council of Australia; ECCO, European Crohn's and Colitis Organization; NICE, National Institute for Health and Clinical Excellence (UK); UC, ulcerative colitis.

Further study is needed to determine which endoscopic features confer the greatest risk of IBD-CRN, and whether limited inflammation or no inflammation is associated with the lowest risk of IBD-CRN. Additional consensus is needed on how to risk-stratify patients and the optimal surveillance intervals for high-, intermediate-, and low-risk patients, as these questions will likely not be answered in prospective studies.

Guidelines Summary

- Patients with the highest risk of IBD-CRN, which includes patients with UC and Crohn's colitis with active extensive disease, PSC, prior history of stricture or dysplasia, or a first-degree relative with CRC before the age of 50, should undergo annual surveillance. Lower-risk patients can undergo surveillance at intervals of every 2 to 5 years.

WHAT IS THE RECOMMENDED TECHNIQUE FOR DYSPLASIA DETECTION?

The goal of surveillance colonoscopy is detection of CRN at its earliest, curable stages. Historically, dysplasia in IBD was thought to be completely flat and endoscopically undetectable, and random biopsies were recommended for dysplasia detection. One prospective study using a 4-quadrant random biopsy protocol every 10 cm calculated that if dysplasia was present in 5% of the colonic mucosa, 33 biopsies were required for histologic detection of dysplasia with 90% confidence.[35] This standard was then endorsed by multiple societies.

Subsequent studies demonstrated that most dysplasia is in fact endoscopically visible, and that random biopsies are overall of low yield in comparison with targeted biopsies of endoscopically abnormal-appearing mucosa.[36–39] Lesion detection is enhanced with dye-based chromoendoscopy using indigo carmine or methylene blue, as demonstrated in multiple RCTs. A recent meta-analysis calculated that chromoendoscopy with targeted biopsy is 8.9 times more likely to detect any dysplasia and 5.2 times more likely to detect nonpolypoid dysplasia than white-light endoscopy with random biopsy.[40] The likelihood to miss dysplasia was 93% lower in colonoscopies performed with chromoendoscopy and targeted biopsy than with white-light and random biopsy, with a number-needed-to-test of 14 to detect 1 additional patient with dysplasia.[40]

Other techniques for image enhanced endoscopy are under investigation, but data currently do not support their routine use.[9,18,41,42] Narrow-band imaging has not demonstrated an increased yield for dysplasia detection during surveillance examinations when compared with chromoendoscopy or white-light endoscopy. Confocal laser endomicroscopy may have a role in the characterization of dysplasia once detected, but additional studies are needed.[42]

At present, chromoendoscopy with targeted biopsies is the surveillance protocol of choice as endorsed by all recent European guidelines (BSG, NICE, ECCO),[1,6,18] with the ECCO group further stating that, "if appropriate expertise for chromoendoscopy is not available, random biopsies should be performed; however this is inferior to chromoendoscopy in the detection rate of neoplastic lesions."[18] Societies in the United States have taken a more conservative approach. The CCFA 2004[3] guidelines endorse chromoendoscopy in appropriately trained endoscopists. The AGA 2010[2] guidelines state that chromoendoscopy with targeted biopsies is a reasonable alternative to white-light endoscopy for endoscopists experienced in this technique. The ACG 2010[4] guidelines state that the natural history of dysplastic lesions detected by chromoendoscopy is unknown, and that it is premature to endorse chromoendoscopy in low-risk patients without longer-term follow-up data. However, chromoendoscopy may be of value for the follow-up of "higher-risk" patients, such as those with known dysplasia or indefinite for dysplasia not undergoing colectomy, and to ensure that detected lesions are adequately resected. The ASGE IBD guidelines are currently under revision, but the recently published ASGE tissue-sampling guidelines[43] endorse chromoendoscopy with targeted biopsies as an option to optimize dysplasia detection with standard white-light endoscopy when the expertise is available.

The BSG, NICE, and ECCO guidelines, while endorsing chromoendoscopy with targeted biopsies as the preferred surveillance technique, further state that the yield of random biopsies of normal-appearing mucosa is low.[1,6,18] The CCA recommends obtaining histologic staging biopsies, as histologic inflammation is a risk factor for IBD-CRN and is used for risk stratification, but do not definitively state that random biopsies are not required.[8] The CCA guidelines recommend that in cases where the yield of chromoendoscopy is reduced, such as with a poor preparation, significant postinflammatory polyps, or significant underlying inflammation, random mucosal sampling may be indicated.[8]

Almost all guidelines that endorse chromoendoscopy do so with the caveat "for appropriately trained endoscopists" or "when the expertise is available." The New Zealand Guidelines Group,[16] which overall endorses the NICE guidelines for surveillance in IBD, states that chromoendoscopy is not available in New Zealand and thus was not considered for the guidelines. It is now incumbent on the training programs and GI professional societies to train endoscopists in the use of chromoendoscopy for the optimal detection of polypoid and nonpolypoid neoplasia.[9] The main utility of chromoendoscopy, as stated in the ECCO consensus document, is its ability to "highlight subtle changes in the architecture of the colonic mucosa,"[18] thus increasing dysplasia detection. Chromoendoscopy can also highlight surface crypt architectural abnormalities, and has been used to guide management of detected lesions.[44,45] Kudo pit-pattern classification can help to characterize detected lesions and their surrounding flat mucosa as having neoplastic (Kudo pit pattern III–V) or non-neoplastic (Kudo pit pattern I or II) architectural changes.[46,47] However, inflammation with regenerative changes can result in Kudo type IIIL or IV pit patterns[48] and, although useful, pit-pattern classification cannot replace histologic evaluation.[49]

Although long-term data on the outcome of dysplasia detected by chromoendoscopy are lacking, the newest guidelines from the BSG, NICE, ECCO, and CCA agree that chromoendoscopy with targeted biopsies maximizes the yield of surveillance colonoscopy for dysplasia detection,[1,6,8,18] which is currently the goal of IBD surveillance. Additional consensus is needed to determine whether there is a role for random biopsies or histologic staging biopsies during chromoendoscopy with targeted biopsy surveillance. Because histologic activity is used to risk-stratify patients in most of the guidelines, it seems prudent to take several biopsies during surveillance colonoscopy even if no targeted biopsies are obtained. How many are required, and whether biopsies should be taken throughout the colon, have yet to be determined.

Guidelines Summary

- The goal of endoscopic surveillance in IBD is to reduce the morbidity and mortality of CRC, by either detecting and resecting dysplasia or detecting CRC at an earlier, potentially curable stage.
- The most recent European and Australian guidelines suggest that to maximize the yield of surveillance colonoscopy for dysplasia detection, chromoendoscopy with targeted biopsies is the surveillance method of choice (**Table 3**). Random biopsies of normal-appearing mucosa are of low yield.
- Histologic staging biopsies may be required for risk stratification of patients.

Table 3
Society guidelines for detected dysplasia

	Visible Dysplastic Lesion, Endoscopically Resectable with Negative Biopsies from Adjacent Mucosa	Visible Dysplastic Lesion, Endoscopically Unresectable or Biopsies from Adjacent Mucosa with Dysplasia	Invisible High-Grade Dysplasia Detected by Random Biopsies	Invisible Low-Grade Dysplasia Detected by Random Biopsies
ECCO,[18] 2013	Surveillance at 3 mo and then yearly, regardless of degree of dysplasia	Colectomy	Confirm by expert GI pathologist Rule out visible lesion with repeat chromoendoscopy surveillance Colectomy if confirmed	Confirm by expert GI pathologist Rule out visible lesion with chromoendoscopy surveillance Consider colectomy vs intensified surveillance with random biopsies
CCA,[8] 2011	Surveillance	Colectomy	Confirm by expert GI pathologist Colectomy	Confirm by expert GI pathologist Multifocal: colectomy vs intensified surveillance at 3–6 mo with chromoendoscopy, then annually Unifocal: consider surgery vs surveillance at 6 mo then annually
BSG,[1] 2010	Surveillance	Colectomy	Not specifically mentioned	Confirm by expert GI pathologist Consider colectomy vs intensified surveillance
ACG,[4] 2010	Surveillance	Colectomy	Confirm by expert GI pathologist Colectomy	Confirm by expert GI pathologist Colectomy vs intensified surveillance
AGA,[2] 2010	Adenoma-like DALM: surveillance (6 mo)	Non-adenoma-like DALM: colectomy	Confirm by expert GI pathologist Colectomy	Confirm by expert GI pathologist Colectomy vs intensified surveillance
ASGE,[5] 2006	Surveillance	DALM: colectomy	Confirm by expert GI pathologist Colectomy	Confirm by expert GI pathologist Multifocal: colectomy Unifocal: consider colectomy vs surveillance at 6 mo then annually
CCFA,[3] 2005				Confirm by expert GI pathologist Multifocal or repetitive: colectomy Unifocal: colectomy; if patient opts for surveillance, then <6-mo intervals recommended

Abbreviations: ACG, American College of Gastroenterology; AGA, American Gastroenterological Society; ASGE, American Society for Gastrointestinal Endoscopy; BSG, British Society for Gastroenterology; CCA, Cancer Council of Australia; CCFA, Crohn's and Colitis Foundation of America; DALM, dysplasia-associated lesion or mass; ECCO, European Crohn's and Colitis Organization; GI, gastrointestinal.

- In situations where the performance of chromoendoscopy is reduced (eg, poor preparation, significant postinflammatory polyps, significant underlying inflammation) or expertise is unavailable, multiple random biopsies with targeted biopsies of white-light detected lesions remains an acceptable alternative.

HOW SHOULD DETECTED DYSPLASIA BE MANAGED?

Older guidelines recommended categorizing detected lesions as sporadic adenomas if found outside an area of known colitis, or as a dysplasia-associated lesion or mass (DALM) if detected within an area of colitis.[9] DALMs were further subcategorized as adenoma-like, if they were raised lesions with an endoscopic appearance of a sporadic adenoma, or non–adenoma-like.[2] Adenoma-like DALMs were amenable to endoscopic resection with close follow-up, whereas non–adenoma-like DALMs were considered an indication for surgery. Colectomy was additionally indicated for high-grade dysplasia detected by random biopsy, and multifocal low-grade dysplasia detected on random biopsy.

Long-term follow-up of endoscopically resected raised dysplastic lesions has been reassuring, with a recent meta-analysis demonstrating a low risk of IBD-CRN following resection of polypoid dysplasia.[50] The use of chromoendoscopy and other image-enhancing techniques not only enhances dysplasia detection, it can also help to delineate lesion borders and facilitate lesion characterization to determine whether a detected lesion is endoscopically resectable or not.[9,44,45]

In this era of image-enhanced endoscopy, a simplified management approach to detect dysplastic lesions is now recommended. Although the terminology is evolving, the newest ECCO consensus guidelines recommend characterizing dysplasia as endoscopically visible or nonvisible.[18] Nonvisible dysplasia refers to dysplasia detected by random biopsy and not associated with an endoscopically visible lesion. According to these ECCO consensus guidelines, well-circumscribed lesions that appear to be endoscopically resectable should be completely resected by an experienced endoscopist, regardless of underlying colitis or grade of dysplasia. If complete resection is achieved with negative biopsies from the flat mucosa immediately adjacent to the polypectomy site, and no dysplasia is found elsewhere in the colon, close endoscopic surveillance, preferably with chromoendoscopy, at 3 months and then at least annually is appropriate. An unresectable lesion or a lesion with dysplasia in the adjacent mucosa is an indication for colectomy. If dysplasia is not associated with a visible lesion, but is found on random biopsy, repeat evaluation with chromoendoscopy by an experienced endoscopist is warranted to assess for a visible and resectable dysplastic lesion and to evaluate for synchronous dysplasia; in this case, random biopsies may be indicated.[18]

These guidelines highlight that the most important feature of well-circumscribed, detected lesions is endoscopic resectability, with confirmation that adjacent mucosa is negative for dysplasia. Older guidelines follow similar recommendations using different terminology.

The definition of endoscopic resectability will continue to evolve. Consensus is needed to standardize the terminology of detected dysplastic lesions and dysplasia detected by random biopsies not associated with an endoscopically visible lesion. Additional consensus is required to determine optimal surveillance after a dysplastic lesion is resected, and how or if the degree of dysplasia should influence the surveillance interval. While endoscopically invisible high-grade dysplasia is universally considered an indication for colectomy, the approach to low-grade dysplasia needs further clarification.

Guidelines Summary

- Endoscopically visible lesions that are well circumscribed and amenable to resection, with no evidence of dysplasia in the surrounding mucosa or elsewhere in the colon on nontargeted biopsies, are appropriate for continued colonoscopic surveillance.
- Endoscopically invisible high-grade dysplasia, detected by random biopsy alone, is an indication for colectomy.
- Societies differ in their recommendations for endoscopically invisible low-grade dysplasia.

SUMMARY

Surveillance colonoscopy is indicated in patients with left-sided or extensive UC, and in patients with Crohn's colitis with involvement of more than 1 colonic segment. The goal of surveillance is to detect dysplasia and to prevent IBD-CRN. Risk factors for IBD-CRN that influence screening and surveillance intervals require further study. To maximize dysplasia detection, European society guidelines endorse chromoendoscopy with targeted biopsies, although societies in the United States have yet to endorse chromoendoscopy as the preferred method for IBD-CRN surveillance. The European guidelines endorsing chromoendoscopy do not require random biopsies of normal-appearing colonic mucosa. However, the role of random biopsies for dysplasia detection needs to be clarified in the setting of inflammation or in areas of pseudopolyps, when the yield of chromoendoscopy may be decreased. Although histologic staging is important for the risk stratification of patients in almost all guidelines, the number of biopsies required and where they should be obtained needs further clarification. Most guidelines agree that well-circumscribed endoscopically detected dysplasia amenable to resection, with no evidence of dysplasia in the surrounding mucosa or elsewhere in the colon, is appropriate for surveillance. However, the definition of endoscopic resectability will continue to evolve, and consensus is needed for both the terminology and the approach to endoscopically visible and nonvisible dysplasia.

REFERENCES

1. Cairns SR, Scholefield JH, Steele RJ, et al. Guidelines for colorectal cancer screening and surveillance in moderate and high risk groups (update from 2002). Gut 2010;59:666–89.
2. Farraye FA, Odze RD, Eaden J, et al. AGA technical review on the diagnosis and management of colorectal neoplasia in inflammatory bowel disease. Gastroenterology 2010;138:746–74, 74.e1–4; [quiz: e12–3].
3. Itzkowitz SH, Present DH. Consensus conference: colorectal cancer screening and surveillance in inflammatory bowel disease. Inflamm Bowel Dis 2005;11: 314–21.
4. Kornbluth A, Sachar DB. Ulcerative colitis practice guidelines in adults: American College Of Gastroenterology, Practice Parameters Committee. Am J Gastroenterol 2010;105:501–23 [quiz: 24].
5. Leighton JA, Shen B, Baron TH, et al. ASGE guideline: endoscopy in the diagnosis and treatment of inflammatory bowel disease. Gastrointest Endosc 2006; 63:558–65.
6. National Institute for Health and Clinical Excellence. Colonoscopic Surveillance for Prevention of Colorectal Cancer in People with Ulcerative Colitis, Crohn's Disease or Adenomas. Clinical Guidelines, No. 118. London 2011.

7. Van Assche G, Dignass A, Bokemeyer B, et al. Second European evidence-based consensus on the diagnosis and management of ulcerative colitis part 3: special situations. J Crohn's Colitis 2012;7:1–33.

8. Cancer Council Australia Colonoscopy Surveillance Working Party. Clinical Practice Guidelines for Surveillance Colonoscopy – in adenoma follow-up; following curative resection of colorectal cancer; and for cancer surveillance in inflammatory bowel disease. Sydney, Australia: Cancer Council Australia; December, 2011. p. 48–62.

9. Rutter MD, Riddell RH. Colorectal dysplasia in inflammatory bowel disease: a clinicopathologic perspective. Clin Gastroenterol Hepatol 2013;12:359–67.

10. Choi PM, Nugent FW, Schoetz DJ Jr, et al. Colonoscopic surveillance reduces mortality from colorectal cancer in ulcerative colitis. Gastroenterology 1993; 105:418–24.

11. Eaden J, Abrams K, Ekbom A, et al. Colorectal cancer prevention in ulcerative colitis: a case-control study. Aliment Pharmacol Ther 2000;14:145–53.

12. Karlen P, Kornfeld D, Brostrom O, et al. Is colonoscopic surveillance reducing colorectal cancer mortality in ulcerative colitis? A population based case control study. Gut 1998;42:711–4.

13. Lashner BA, Kane SV, Hanauer SB. Colon cancer surveillance in chronic ulcerative colitis: historical cohort study. Am J Gastroenterol 1990;85:1083–7.

14. Lutgens MW, Oldenburg B, Siersema PD, et al. Colonoscopic surveillance improves survival after colorectal cancer diagnosis in inflammatory bowel disease. Br J Cancer 2009;101:1671–5.

15. Collins PD, Mpofu C, Watson AJ, et al. Strategies for detecting colon cancer and/or dysplasia in patients with inflammatory bowel disease. Cochrane Database Syst Rev 2006;(2):CD000279.

16. New Zealand Guidelines Group. Guidance on surveillance for people at increased risk of colorectal cancer 2011. Wellington (New Zealand): New Zealand Guidelines Group; 2011.

17. Rufo PA, Denson LA, Sylvester FA, et al. Health supervision in the management of children and adolescents with IBD: NASPGHAN recommendations. J Pediatr Gastroenterol Nutr 2012;55:93–108.

18. Annese V, Daperno M, Rutter MD, et al. European evidence based consensus for endoscopy in inflammatory bowel disease. J Crohn's Colitis 2013;7:982–1018.

19. Lichtenstein GR, Hanauer SB, Sandborn WJ, Practice Parameters Committee of American College of Gastroenterology. Management of Crohn's disease in adults. Am J Gastroenterol 2009;104:465–83 [quiz: 464, 484].

20. Eaden JA, Abrams KR, Mayberry JF. The risk of colorectal cancer in ulcerative colitis: a meta-analysis. Gut 2001;48:526–35.

21. Rutter MD, Saunders BP, Wilkinson KH, et al. Thirty-year analysis of a colonoscopic surveillance program for neoplasia in ulcerative colitis. Gastroenterology 2006;130:1030–8.

22. Lutgens MW, Vleggaar FP, Schipper ME, et al. High frequency of early colorectal cancer in inflammatory bowel disease. Gut 2008;57:1246–51.

23. Baars JE, Kuipers EJ, van Haastert M, et al. Age at diagnosis of inflammatory bowel disease influences early development of colorectal cancer in inflammatory bowel disease patients: a nationwide, long-term survey. J Gastroenterol 2012;47:1308–22.

24. Beaugerie L, Svrcek M, Seksik P, et al. Risk of colorectal high-grade dysplasia and cancer in a prospective observational cohort of patients with inflammatory bowel disease. Gastroenterology 2013;145:166–75.e8.

25. Jess T, Rungoe C, Peyrin-Biroulet L. Risk of colorectal cancer in patients with ulcerative colitis: a meta-analysis of population-based cohort studies. Clin Gastroenterol Hepatol 2012;10:639–45.
26. Soetikno RM, Lin OS, Heidenreich PA, et al. Increased risk of colorectal neoplasia in patients with primary sclerosing cholangitis and ulcerative colitis: a meta-analysis. Gastrointest Endosc 2002;56:48–54.
27. Ekbom A, Helmick C, Zack M, et al. Ulcerative colitis and colorectal cancer. A population-based study. N Engl J Med 1990;323:1228–33.
28. Soderlund S, Brandt L, Lapidus A, et al. Decreasing time-trends of colorectal cancer in a large cohort of patients with inflammatory bowel disease. Gastroenterology 2009;136:1561–7 [quiz: 1818–9].
29. Rutter M, Saunders B, Wilkinson K, et al. Severity of inflammation is a risk factor for colorectal neoplasia in ulcerative colitis. Gastroenterology 2004;126:451–9.
30. Rubin DT, Huo D, Kinnucan JA, et al. Inflammation is an independent risk factor for colonic neoplasia in patients with ulcerative colitis: a case-control study. Clin Gastroenterol Hepatol 2013;11:1601–8.e4.
31. Gupta RB, Harpaz N, Itzkowitz S, et al. Histologic inflammation is a risk factor for progression to colorectal neoplasia in ulcerative colitis: a cohort study. Gastroenterology 2007;133:1099–105 [quiz: 340–1].
32. Askling J, Dickman PW, Karlen P, et al. Family history as a risk factor for colorectal cancer in inflammatory bowel disease. Gastroenterology 2001;120:1356–62.
33. Thomas T, Abrams KA, Robinson RJ, et al. Meta-analysis: cancer risk of low-grade dysplasia in chronic ulcerative colitis. Aliment Pharmacol Ther 2007;25:657–68.
34. Rutter MD, Saunders BP, Wilkinson KH, et al. Cancer surveillance in longstanding ulcerative colitis: endoscopic appearances help predict cancer risk. Gut 2004;53:1813–6.
35. Rubin CE, Haggitt RC, Burmer GC, et al. DNA aneuploidy in colonic biopsies predicts future development of dysplasia in ulcerative colitis. Gastroenterology 1992;103:1611–20.
36. Blonski W, Kundu R, Lewis J, et al. Is dysplasia visible during surveillance colonoscopy in patients with ulcerative colitis? Scand J Gastroenterol 2008;43:698–703.
37. Rubin DT, Rothe JA, Hetzel JT, et al. Are dysplasia and colorectal cancer endoscopically visible in patients with ulcerative colitis? Gastrointest Endosc 2007;65:998–1004.
38. Rutter MD, Saunders BP, Wilkinson KH, et al. Most dysplasia in ulcerative colitis is visible at colonoscopy. Gastrointest Endosc 2004;60:334–9.
39. van den Broek FJ, Stokkers PC, Reitsma JB, et al. Random biopsies taken during colonoscopic surveillance of patients with longstanding ulcerative colitis: low yield and absence of clinical consequences. Am J Gastroenterol 2011. [Epub ahead of print].
40. Soetikno R, Subramanian V, Kaltenbach T, et al. The detection of nonpolypoid (flat and depressed) colorectal neoplasms in patients with inflammatory bowel disease. Gastroenterology 2013;144:1349–52, 1352.e1–6.
41. East JE. Colonoscopic cancer surveillance in inflammatory bowel disease: what's new beyond random biopsy? Clin Endosc 2012;45:274–7.
42. Murthy SK, Kiesslich R. Evolving endoscopic strategies for detection and treatment of neoplastic lesions in inflammatory bowel disease. Gastrointest Endosc 2013;77:351–9.

43. Committee ASoP, Sharaf RN, Shergill AK, et al. Endoscopic mucosal tissue sampling. Gastrointest Endosc 2013;78:216–24.
44. Hurlstone DP, Sanders DS, Atkinson R, et al. Endoscopic mucosal resection for flat neoplasia in chronic ulcerative colitis: can we change the endoscopic management paradigm? Gut 2007;56:838–46.
45. Smith LA, Baraza W, Tiffin N, et al. Endoscopic resection of adenoma-like mass in chronic ulcerative colitis using a combined endoscopic mucosal resection and cap assisted submucosal dissection technique. Inflamm Bowel Dis 2008; 14:1380–6.
46. Kiesslich R, Fritsch J, Holtmann M, et al. Methylene blue-aided chromoendoscopy for the detection of intraepithelial neoplasia and colon cancer in ulcerative colitis. Gastroenterology 2003;124:880–8.
47. Kudo S, Rubio CA, Teixeira CR, et al. Pit pattern in colorectal neoplasia: endoscopic magnifying view. Endoscopy 2001;33:367–73.
48. Hata K, Watanabe T, Motoi T, et al. Pitfalls of pit pattern diagnosis in ulcerative colitis-associated dysplasia. Gastroenterology 2004;126:374–6.
49. Thorlacius H, Toth E. Role of chromoendoscopy in colon cancer surveillance in inflammatory bowel disease. Inflamm Bowel Dis 2007;13:911–7.
50. Wanders LK, Dekker E, Pullens B, et al. Cancer risk after resection of polypoid dysplasia in patients with longstanding ulcerative colitis: a meta-analysis. Clin Gastroenterol Hepatol 2014;12:756–64.

An Atlas of the Nonpolypoid Colorectal Neoplasms in Inflammatory Bowel Disease

Roy Soetikno, MD[a],*, Silvia Sanduleanu, MD, PhD[b], Tonya Kaltenbach, MD[a]

KEYWORDS

- Inflammatory bowel disease • Nonpolypoid colorectal neoplasms
- Colorectal cancer • Chromoendoscopy • Surveillance colonoscopy

KEY POINTS

- Patients with inflammatory bowel disease (IBD) have an increased risk of colorectal cancer (CRC).
- Studies suggest that the current standard of colonoscopy surveillance with random biopsies to detect dysplasia in IBD patients is inadequate.
- With the use of current knowledge, technology and techniques most dysplasia in IBD patients is visible during colonoscopy.
- Data and guidelines now support the use of chromoendoscopy with targeted biopsy in the detection of dysplasia and/or colorectal cancer in patients with colitic IBD.

INTRODUCTION

The role of endoscopy in the management of patients with inflammatory bowel disease (IBD) is well established. However, recent data have shown significant limitations in the effectiveness of the use of colonoscopy to prevent colorectal cancer (CRC) in patients with IBD colitis. The current standard using random biopsy appeared to be largely ineffective in detecting the nonpolypoid colorectal neoplasms (NP-CRN). Data using chromoendoscopy with targeted biopsy, however, showed a significant improvement when used to detect dysplasia, the best predictor of colorectal cancer risk. The purpose of this monograph is to provide the medical profession with a useful and organized series of images showing the superficial elevated, flat, and depressed colorectal neoplasms and their appearance after the application of the technique of chromoendoscopy.

[a] Veterans Affairs Palo Alto, Stanford University School of Medicine, 3801 Miranda Avenue, GI 111, Palo Alto, CA 94304, USA; [b] Division of Gastroenterology and Hepatology, GROW, School for Oncology and Developmental Biology, Maastricht University Medical Center, Postbox 5800, 6202 AZ, Maastricht, The Netherlands
* Corresponding author. Veterans Affairs Palo Alto, Stanford University, 3801 Miranda Avenue, Palo Alto, CA.
E-mail address: giendo@me.com

Gastrointest Endoscopy Clin N Am 24 (2014) 483–520
http://dx.doi.org/10.1016/j.giec.2014.04.003
1052-5157/14/$ – see front matter Published by Elsevier Inc.

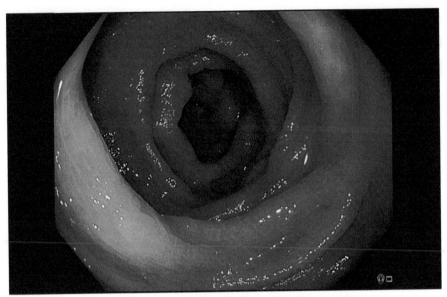

Fig. 1. Endoscopic view of nonpolypoid colorectal neoplasm.

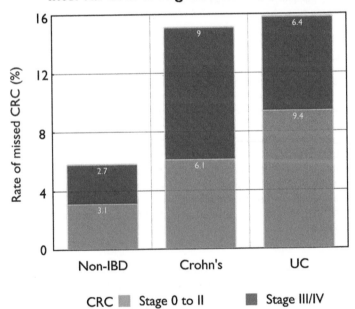

Fig. 2. Current surveillance against CRC is associated with a high risk of interval cancer. In a study of 55,000 Medicare patients diagnosed with CRC, patients with IBD were 3 times more likely to have had a recent colonoscopy than patients without IBD. A significant fraction (15%) of the IBD patients who were diagnosed with CRC had undergone surveillance colonoscopy in the prior 3 years. Note that many of these cancers were advanced. These data indicate that the standard method used during surveillance colonoscopy, namely the random biopsy technique, is inadequate.[1]

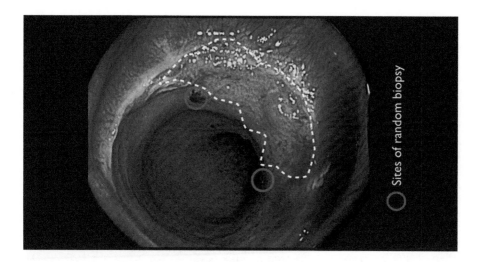

Fig. 3. Random biopsy without interpreting what is being viewed is not effective. This example shows that random biopsy of the colon to detect and diagnose dysplasia has a high miss rate.[2] In this patient, random biopsies were taken from the circled areas, as shown by the blood. Unfortunately the neoplasia (*encircled by the dashed line*) was not biopsied. Note that the high-definition adult colonoscope was used, and the lesion was not detected. High definition increases the resolution of the image. For example, high definition captures at least 720 pixels from top to bottom (with most capturing 1080 pixels), whereas standard definition captures 480 pixels. What is needed, however, is not only increased resolution, but also improved contrast between dysplastic and nondysplastic mucosa. If the dysplasia can be highlighted or colored distinctly, its detection and diagnosis may be easier.

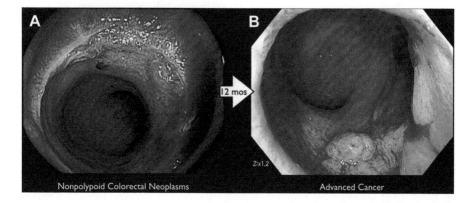

Fig. 4. An example of an interval cancer in a patient with ulcerative colitis. This patient was referred to the authors 1 year after image (*A*) was taken. He presented for staging endoscopic ultrasonography after a repeat surveillance showed an ulcerated mass lesion (*B*). The lesion had become an advanced cancer. He underwent a total proctocolectomy. T2, N2 poorly differentiated carcinoma was found.

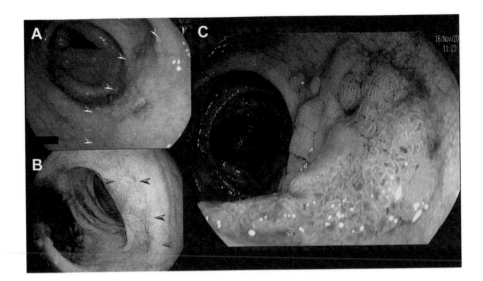

Fig. 5. Chromoendoscopy facilitates visualization of NP-CRN. (*A*) The lesion was difficult to appreciate with high-definition white-light endoscopy. A possible flat lesion was noted retrospectively, as shown by the white arrowheads. (*B*) The patient presented for follow-up 6 months later. A possible superficial elevated lesion was noted (*blue arrowheads*). (*C*) After application of dilute indigo carmine, the lesion and its borders were easily detected.

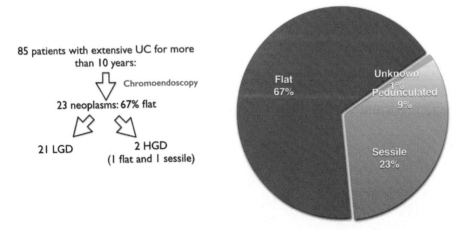

Fig. 6. NP-CRN are relatively common in patients with long-standing ulcerative colitis. Jaramillo and colleagues studied the yield of performing chromoendoscopy in patients with extensive and long-standing ulcerative colitis, and found that most neoplasms were flat. The detection of these superficial elevated, flat, or depressed neoplasms, however, poses a special challenge because the background mucosa is often scarred or inflamed.[3] HGD, high-grade dysplasia; LGD, low-grade dysplasia; UC, ulcerative colitis.

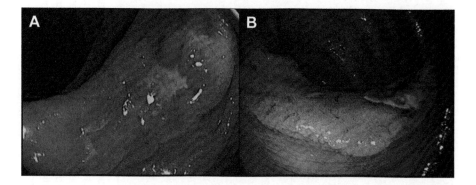

Fig. 7. Most colorectal neoplasms in colitic IBD are believed to be visible. A lesion might be considered an "invisible" neoplasm because it was not recognized during the examination.[4] The lesion shown in (A), despite being photographed en face, was not recognized as a superficial elevated lesion with an ulcer. The endoscopist missed the lesion again during a repeat surveillance colonoscopy 5 months later, which was performed to survey a pedunculated polyp resection site. The patient, who has long-standing Crohn's colitis, presented to the authors 14 months later for surveillance colonoscopy. A similar-appearing lesion was easily detected using chromoendoscopy (B). Understanding the appearance of the NP-CRN and the signs of its presence are critical to performing an efficacious colonoscopy.

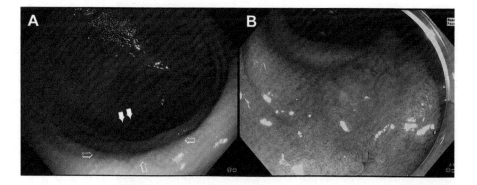

Fig. 8. Understanding the techniques useful to visualize NP-CRN is important, as NP-CRN in patients with colitic IBD can be very difficult to detect. This patient with Crohn's colitis had endoscopic mucosal resection (EMR) of a superficial elevated NP-CRN. The pathology of the lesion showed low-grade dysplasia (LGD). However, the biopsies of the surrounding mucosa also showed LGD. Thus, he was referred for further evaluation. In (A), a slightly more reddish mucosa was seen (*open arrows*). Chromoendoscopy with indigo carmine was used to delineate the border of the lesion (B). The lesion had a distinct border. It was completely endoscopically resected and found to be LGD. Note that a distal attachment cap was required to push the fold (*double solid arrows*) to examine the area proximal to the fold.[5]

NOMENCLATURE

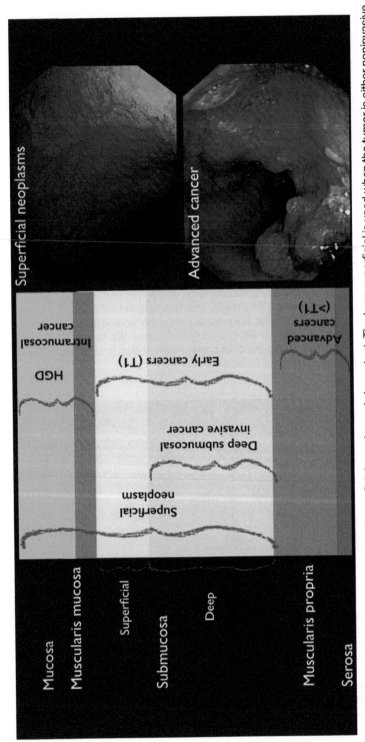

Fig. 9. Understanding the nomenclature of superficial neoplasms is important. The term superficial is used when the tumor is either noninvasive appearing or small. Superficial includes noncancer neoplasms, and mucosal and submucosal invasive cancers. A subset of superficial cancers that appear to have a significant invasion into the submucosa is called massive submucosal invasive cancer. Matsuda and colleagues suggested that the presence of redness, firm consistency, expansion, and deep depression are important findings of deeply submucosal invasive cancer.[6] In the upper image, the neoplastic lesion appeared benign and limited to the mucosa. It has none of the findings of deeply submucosal invasion. In the lower image, the lesion was large, and invaded deeply into the wall. The lesion was red, firm appearing, full, and had deep depression. The lesion in the upper image may be removable by endoscopy, whereas surgery would be required for the lesion in the lower image.

Macroscopic Classification of Superficial Colorectal Neoplasms (Type 0)

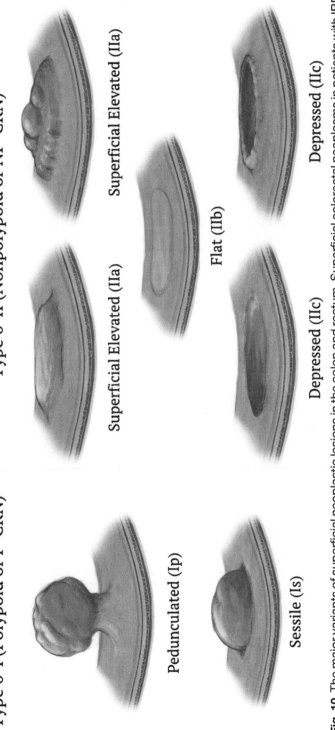

Fig. 10. The major variants of superficial neoplastic lesions in the colon and rectum. Superficial colorectal neoplasms in patients with IBD can be described.[7,8] Lesions are classified as protruding (polypoid) and nonprotruding (nonpolypoid). Polypoid neoplasms may be further divided into pedunculated (0-Ip) or sessile (0-Is). Nonpolypoid lesions can be divided into slightly elevated/table top (IIa), depressed (IIc), or completely flat (IIb). An international group of IBD experts, endoscopists, pathologists, and methodologists who gathered in San Francisco in March 2014 (SCENIC Consensus) suggested that the current classifications for IBD patients should also include: (1) description of an ulcer, if present, within the lesion; and (2) description of the border of the lesion, especially if it cannot be recognized.[9]

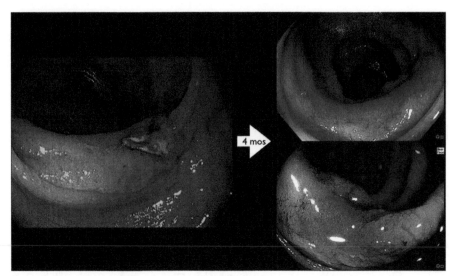

Fig. 11. The presence of an ulcer within a lesion needs to be characterized. A 4-cm superficial elevated neoplasm in a patient with long-standing Crohn's colitis with a 7-mm ulcer is shown. The ulcer appeared benign; its edge was not full and its base did not appear deep or nodular. The patient elected to have a slightly delayed endoscopic resection, rather than an immediate surgery. He was treated with a short course (2 months) of oral steroids. The ulcer resolved following escalation of medical therapy, and the circumscribed superficial elevated lesion was treated with endoscopic resection. The pathology indicated LGD. The presence of an ulcer within a lesion, however, may indicate carcinomatous degeneration.

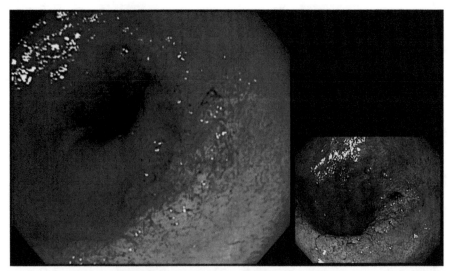

Fig. 12. The absence of the border of the lesion needs to be characterized. This ill-defined nodular, friable, irregular surface was seen in the rectum during surveillance examination. Even following the application of chromoendoscopy, the border remained unable to be visualized. Such a lesion is not amenable to endoscopic resection, and targeted biopsy should be performed. A tattoo of the area for marking was made, and the patient was referred for surgical evaluation.

SIGNS OF NONPOLYPOID COLORECTAL NEOPLASMS IN IBD

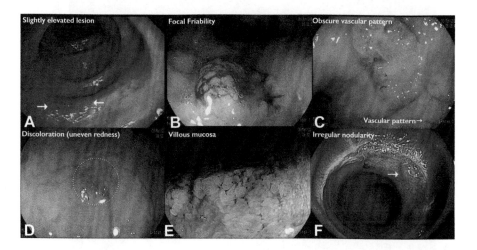

Fig. 13. Signs of NP-CRN in colitic IBD. The detection of flat and depressed neoplasms in colitic IBD, unlike the detection of polypoid neoplasms, relies primarily on the recognition of subtle changes in the mucosa. The subtle findings require constant awareness by the endoscopist for areas that appear to be slightly different than the background in color, pattern, or level. (A) Nonpolypoid lesions typically have a slightly elevated appearance that can often be recognized by a deformity on the colon wall (*arrows*). (B) Occasionally there may be spontaneous hemorrhage on the surface. The surface may be friable. (C) Obscure vascular pattern or (D) increased erythema (*within circle*) may suggest a lesion is present, in that these lesions may disturb the mucosal vascular network. The surface pattern may show (E) villous features or (F) irregular nodularity (*arrow*).

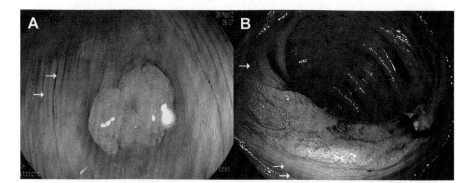

Fig. 14. Interruption of the innominate grooves can alert the endoscopist to the presence of NP-CRN. Innominate grooves, on histology, are mucosal areas where several crypts open into one central crypt. (A) On endoscopy, they are visible in normal colonic mucosa and nonneoplastic lesions (*arrows*), whereas they are interrupted in neoplastic lesions. (B) These areas can be better observed following the application of dye, such as indigo carmine, as the dye pools into the grooves and makes them appear as blue lines (*arrows*).

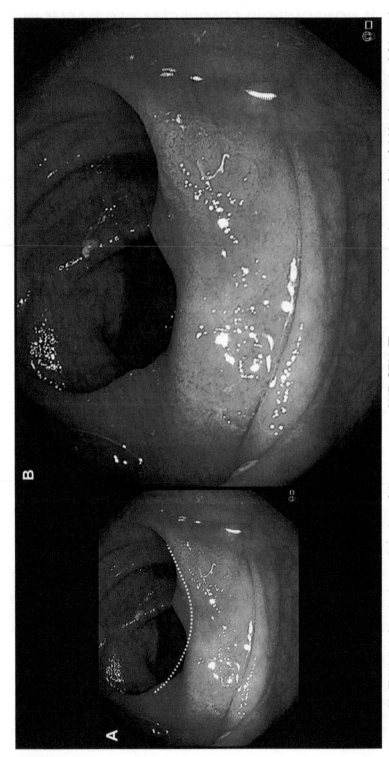

Fig. 15. (*A*, *B*) Wall deformity is another sign of the presence of NP-CRN. The expected natural curve of the fold is shown in *A* (*dotted line*). In this case, the wall was deformed. A large superficial flat neoplasm was the cause of this deformity.

PHOTODOCUMENTATION

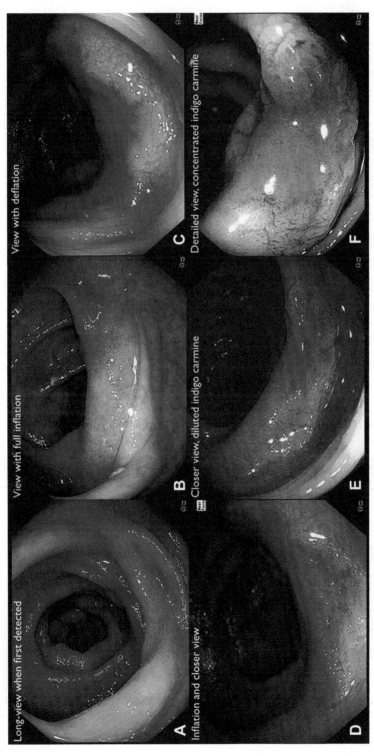

Fig. 16. General to detailed visualization of a superficial elevated neoplasm and its imaging documentation. Examination of a lesion to understand the significance of its detail is a fluid stepwise process. For example, (A) on detection, the lesion is first viewed in a long view, to understand and evaluate its relative size, shape, and location. The lesion is then examined with varying expansion of the colon. Increasing (B) or decreasing (C) air insufflation may help improve visualization of a flat or depressed lesion. (D) Closer view permits detailed examination of the vessel and surface pattern. (E, F) Application of indigo carmine dye further enhances the borders of the lesion and the details of the morphology and surface pattern.

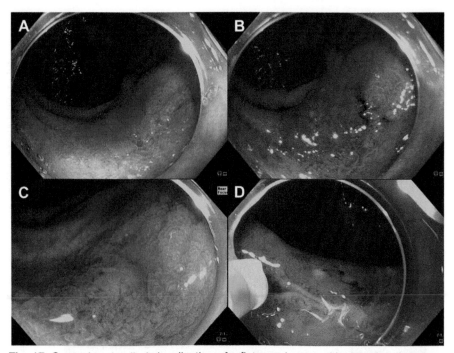

Fig. 17. General to detailed visualization of a flat neoplasm and its imaging documentation, illustrating the use of a translucent distal attachment device (cap) in the detailed view and understanding of the lesion. Documentation of the lesion is best performed by taking an overview (long-shot) picture, before close-up pictures are taken (*A, B, C*). In (*A*), the lesion is inspected using high definition white light. In (*B*), narrow-band imaging (NBI) was used to visualize the surface and microvessel patterns. In (*C*), indigo carmine was used to determine the margin of the lesion. Pit-pattern characterization of the lesion using either NBI or indigo carmine is generally not useful. Detailed imaging of the lesion is critical for its complete resection. (*D*) A circumferential cut was performed to isolate the lesion before its snaring.

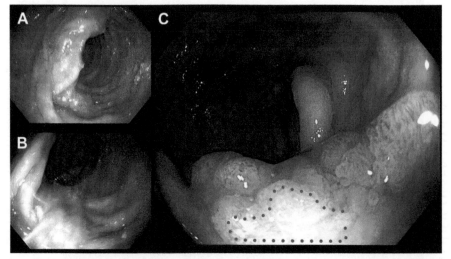

Fig. 18. (*A–C*) White-out (halation) can impair adequate viewing and interpretation. There is a blurred effect around the edges of the area highlighted caused by reflection and scattering of light.

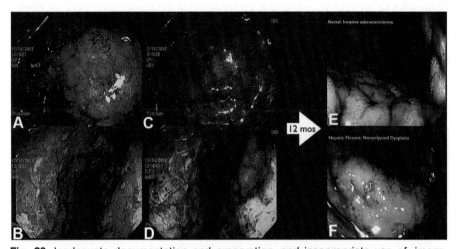

	Purpose	Long-view	Close-view
Peak	Prevent white out during close view	Dark (Bad)	Great **USE**
Average or Auto	Provide ideal light for long view	Great **USE**	Halation (Bad)

Fig. 19. Appropriate setting of the iris is important. The iris function on endoscope processors adjusts the distribution of light, and is generally sufficient to adjust brightness.

- Auto: The brightness is adjusted based on the brightest part of the central part and the average brightness of the periphery part.
- Peak: The brightness is adjusted based on the brightest part of the endoscopic image.

Fig. 20. Inadequate documentation and preparation, and inappropriate use of, image-enhanced endoscopy. A picture is worth a thousand words, except when the picture is not adequate. In this case, only close-up images were taken (*A–F*). In addition, surveillance for IBD dysplasia must be performed in patients with inactive disease, with bowel preparation of adequate quality and the appropriate imaging and tools. A surveillance colonoscopy with random biopsies was performed with the aid of NBI in this 41-year-old patient with long-standing Crohn's colitis and primary sclerosing cholangitis (*A, B*). Importantly the images show severe disease inactivity and inadequate bowel preparation. NBI, which has not been shown to provide any benefit for detection of dysplasia when compared with white light or chromoendoscopy, was used (*C, D*). Random biopsies were performed, which showed severe chronic active colitis with focal LGD in the right colon, and moderate chronic active colitis in the transverse and left colon. No biopsies were taken of the rectum. One year later, a repeat colonoscopy was performed in the setting of less active disease using chromoendoscopy with targeted biopsy. Targeted biopsy showed (*E*) an invasive low-grade adenocarcinoma in the rectum and (*F*) a nonpolypoid dysplastic lesion in the hepatic flexure.

GENERAL PRINCIPLES

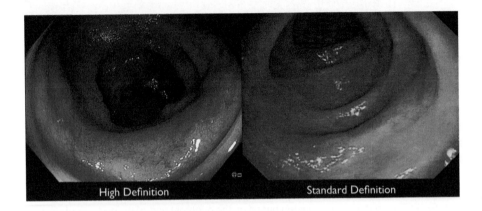

Fig. 21. High-definition white-light imaging is superior to standard-definition white-light imaging for surveillance of dysplasia in the detection of dysplasia and/or CRC in patients with colitic IBD. Surveillance using high-definition colonoscopy detected significantly more patients with dysplasia (prevalence ratio 2.3, 95% confidence interval [CI] 1.03–5.11) and detected significantly more endoscopically visible dysplasia (risk ratio 3.4, 95% CI 1.3–8.9).[10]

Chromoendoscopy with targeted biopsy leads to increased efficacy compared to white light colonoscopy

- Leads to 7% (95% CI: 3.3 to 10.3%) increase in the detection of dysplasia/patient

- NNT to find another patient with at least one dysplasia: 14.3 (range 9.7 to 30.3)

- Likelihood to find any dysplasia: Odds ratio: 8.9 (95% CI: 3.4 to 23)

- Likelihood to find flat dysplasia: Odds ratio 5.2 (95% CI: 1.7 to 15.9)

Box. 1. Chromoendoscopy with targeted biopsy leads to increased efficacy of surveillance. In a meta-analysis of 6 clinical trials comparing chromoendoscopy with white-light endoscopy, chromoendoscopy detected additional dysplasia in 7% of patients in comparison with white-light endoscopy. The number needed to treat (NNT) to find another patient with at least 1 dysplasia was 14. Chromoendoscopy with targeted biopsy increased the likelihood of detecting any dysplasia by 9 times when compared with white light, and the likelihood of detecting nonpolypoid dysplasia was 5 times higher. (*Data from* Soetikno R, Subramanian V, Kaltenbach T, et al. The detection of nonpolypoid (flat and depressed) colorectal neoplasms in patients with inflammatory bowel disease. Gastroenterology 2013;144(7):1349–52.)

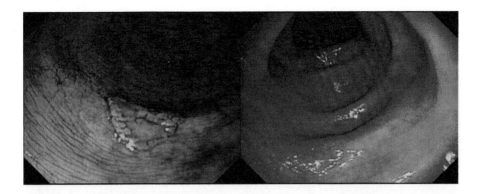

Fig. 22. Standard definition chromoendoscopy is superior to standard definition white light imaging in the detection of dysplasia and/or CRC in patients with colitic IBD. A meta-analysis of 8 studies that included a total of 785 patients with IBD, 82 (10.4%) of whom were later found to have dysplasia and 7, cancer (0.89%), showed superiority in the use of chromoendoscopy (*left*) when compared with white light (*right*):

1. Detected significantly more patients with dysplasia: incremental yield 6%, 95% CI 2.8% to 9.2%
2. Detected significantly more patients with endoscopically visible dysplasia: incremental yield 7%, 95% CI 3.0% to 10.0%
3. Detected significantly more dysplasia: incremental yield 15%, 95% CI 5.0% to 24.0%.

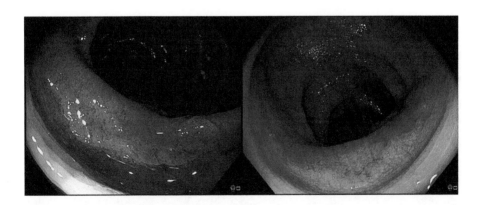

Fig. 23. High definition with indigo carmine is superior to high definition white light in the detection of dysplasia and/or colorectal cancer in patients with colitic IBD.

1. Detected significantly more patients with dysplasia, 21.3% (16/75) versus 9.3% (7/75), incremental yield 12% ($P = .007$)
2. Detected significantly more endoscopically visible dysplasia, 100% (22/22) versus 45.4% (10/22), incremental yield 16% ($P = .004$)
3. Detected significantly more patients with nonpolypoid dysplastic lesions, 9.3% versus 1.3%, incremental yield 8% ($P = .011$).[11]

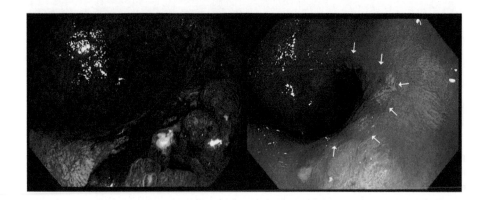

Fig. 24. High definition NBI is not superior to high-definition white light in the detection of dysplasia in IBD patients. Two studies on the performance of surveillance colonoscopy with a high definition colonoscope were performed to compare NBI with white light. A total of 160 patients with IBD, 21 (13.1%) of whom were later found to have dysplasia and none, cancer, were studied. The use of NBI, compared with white light, did not lead to significant differences in the number of patients who were found to have any dysplasia. In fact, the use of NBI led to decreased detection of dysplastic lesions.[12,13] The first generation of NBI was used in the studies and in this image. Note that the use of NBI caused the image to become quite dark. On biopsy of the depressed area (*arrows*), high-grade dysplasia (HGD) was found.

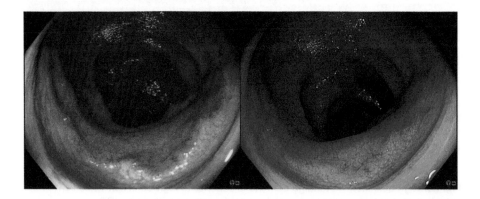

Fig. 25. A large, superficial, elevated lesion was imaged using the latest generation of NBI. The image was still somewhat dark.

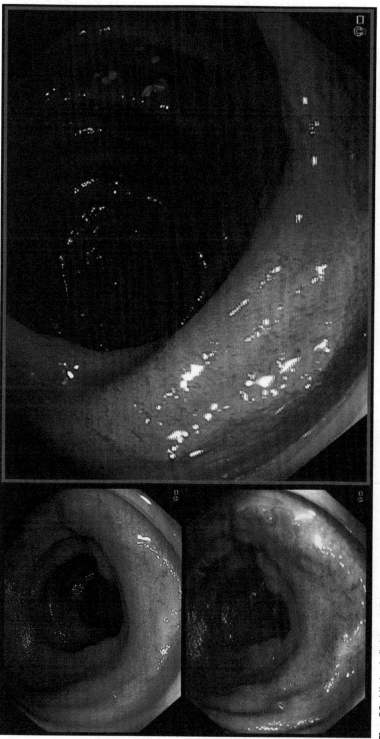

Fig. 26. High-definition NBI is not superior to high-definition chromoendoscopy. There has been interest to use NBI in lieu of chromoendoscopy in IBD surveillance. Four studies on surveillance colonoscopy with high-definition colonoscopy have been performed to compare chromoendoscopy with NBI. NBI was not shown to be advantageous. In fact, surveillance with chromoendoscopy showed a 6% (95% CI −1.4% to 14.2%) higher yield in the detection of patients with dysplasia in comparison with NBI, although the difference did not reach statistical significance.

TECHNIQUE OF CHROMOENDOSCOPY WITH TARGETED BIOPSY

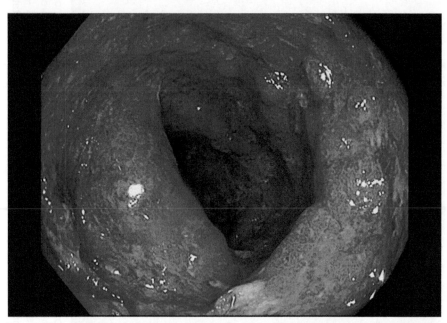

Fig. 27. The disease should be in remission before surveillance is undertaken. Active colitis causes changes in mucosal color, texture, and vascularity that can be extremely difficult to distinguish from nonpolypoid neoplasia. Furthermore, mucosal inflammation and regeneration can cause cytologic changes that can mimic dysplasia.

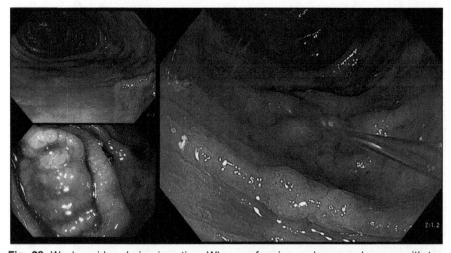

Fig. 28. Wash residue during insertion. When performing a chromoendoscopy with targeted biopsy, irrigate the colon of debris with water while intubating to the cecum. Any remaining residue should be meticulously washed and suctioned before the application of chromoendoscopy. Chromoendoscopy begins once one reaches the cecum and the colonoscope is withdrawn. Performing chromoendoscopy when the colon is dirty is very difficult: when the blue dye mixes with the bilious stool, it turns green.

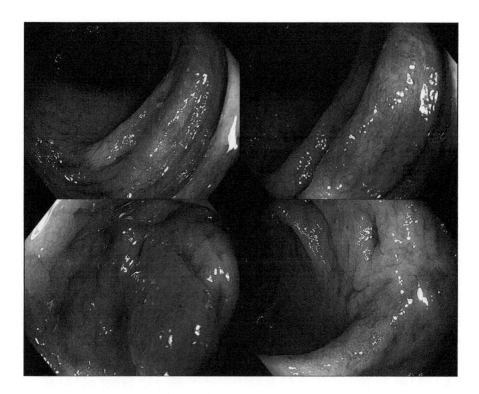

Fig. 29. Target biopsies of abnormal or suspicious areas. Most dysplasia is visible and, thus, biopsies should be targeted. Rather than taking random biopsies, the endoscopist compares the color, pattern of the pits, glands, and, when visible, the microvessels to the background mucosa to target biopsies to abnormal-appearing areas.

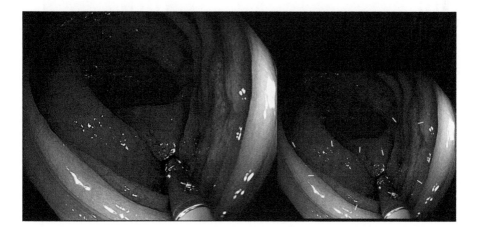

Fig. 30. Evaluate lesions thoroughly. A biopsy forceps was used to investigate part of the large, superficial, elevated lesion that lay behind the fold. The colon was slightly deflated as the forceps was used to expose the proximal side of the lesion.

Algorithm of pancolonic chromoendoscopy and targeted biopsy, and management of detected superficial colorectal lesions

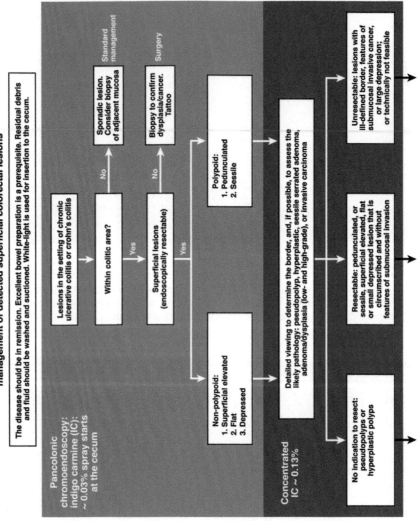

The disease should be in remission. Excellent bowel preparation is a prerequisite. Residual debris and fluid should be washed and suctioned. White-light is used for insertion to the cecum.

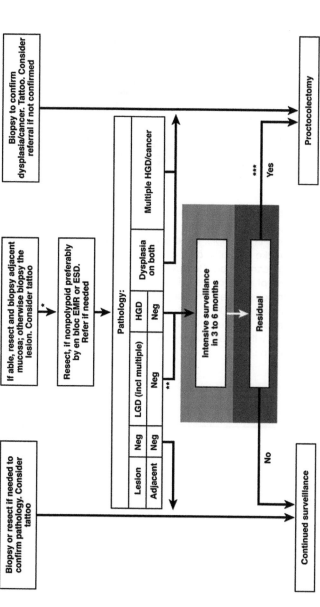

Fig. 31. An algorithm to detect, diagnose, and treat colorectal neoplasms in patients with colitic IBD using chromoendoscopy and targeted biopsy. (*From* Soetikno R, Subramanian V, Kaltenbach T, et al. The detection of nonpolypoid (flat and depressed) colorectal neoplasms in patients with inflammatory bowel disease. Gastroenterology 2013;144(7):1349–52; with permission.)

Concentration of Indigo Carmine used in IBD patients

Purpose of IEE	Mixture	Depth of blue
Detection	2 Ampules with 250 mL of water	
Detailed Viewing	1 Ampule with 25 mL of water	
Submucosal Injection	10 Drops with 100 mL of saline	

Fig. 32. Using high-definition instruments, image-enhanced endoscopy (IEE) is performed with indigo carmine using 3 different concentrations. Varying the concentration is important, depending on the indication. For example, if the solution is too concentrated when spraying the entire colon, it can make the colon dark and impair inspection. The corollary is when selectively spraying indigo carmine on a lesion for detailed inspection the solution is too weak, in which case it does not enhance visualization or contrast. When resecting a lesion, the authors perform submucosal injection using a dilution of indigo carmine and saline (10 drops of indigo carmine with 100 mL of normal saline). (*From* Soetikno R, Subramanian V, Kaltenbach T, et al. The detection of nonpolypoid (flat and depressed) colorectal neoplasms in patients with inflammatory bowel disease. Gastroenterology 2013;144(7):1349–52; with permission.)

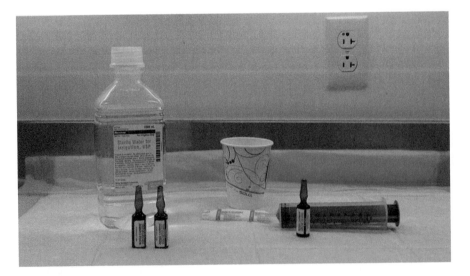

Fig. 33. Mixing of indigo carmine for chromoendoscopy throughout the colon. The forward wash jet solution is made combining 2 ampules of 5 mL of 0.8% indigo carmine with 250 mL of water.

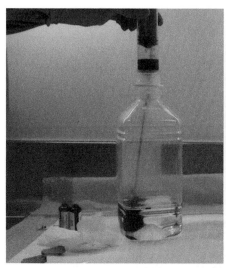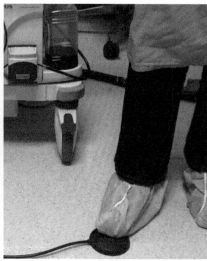

Fig. 34. Equipment for detection of NP-CRN in IBD. After complete insertion of the colonoscope, examination with chromoendoscopy begins in the cecum and proceeds methodically. During withdrawal, each segment is sprayed and carefully inspected. Indigo carmine is spray diluted (~0.03%) through the forward wash jet. For optimal application and efficiency, the foot wash pump is used for spraying, and the spray is targeted to the antigravity wall of the colon. Any excess dye that pools is suctioned so that a thin layer remains and the mucosa is not obscured by blue pools. The lumen is expanded and collapsed with air insufflation and suctioning during chromoendoscopy examination.

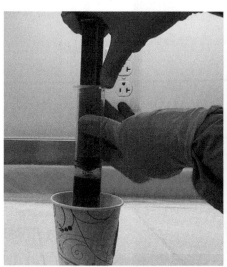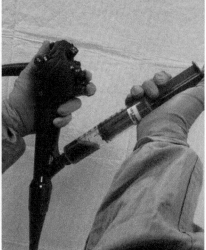

Fig. 35. Detailed viewing. When lesions or possible lesions are identified, more concentrated indigo carmine (0.13%, 5 mL ampule of indigo carmine with 25 mL water) is applied with a syringe via the biopsy channel to better delineate the lesion extent and the mucosal detail.

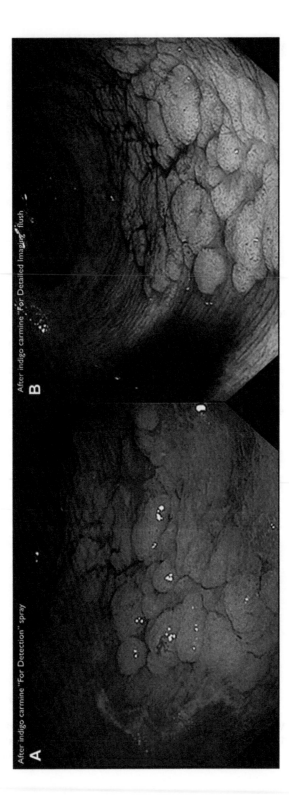

Fig. 36. Lesion identification technique of chromoendoscopy. (*A*) Using a high definition colonoscope, dilute indigo carmine is applied using the forward wash jet. (*B*) When lesions are identified, more concentrated indigo carmine is applied via the biopsy channel to better delineate the lesion extent and the mucosal detail. Targeted biopsies are then taken of the lesion. Biopsies are also taken around the lesion to exclude flat, invisible dysplasia, which would render it endoscopically unresectable.

Pit-pattern classification

Type	Schematic	Endoscopic	Description	Suggested Pathology	Ideal Treatment
I	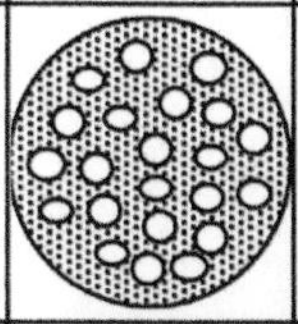	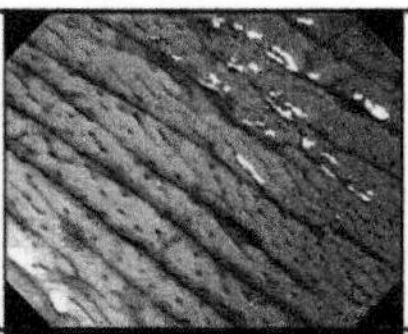	Round pits.	Non-neoplastic.	Endoscopic or none.
II	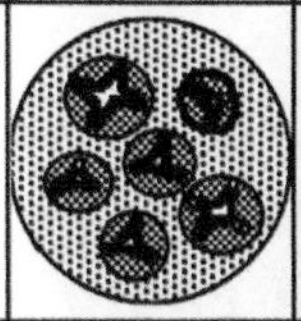	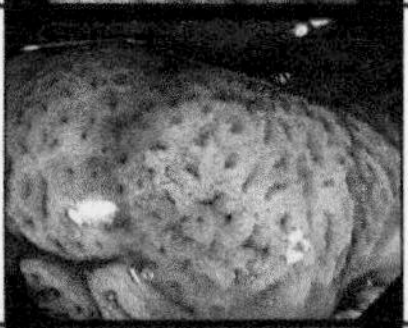	Stellar or papillary pits.	Non-neoplastic.	Endoscopic or none.
IIIs	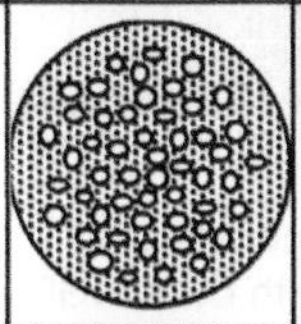	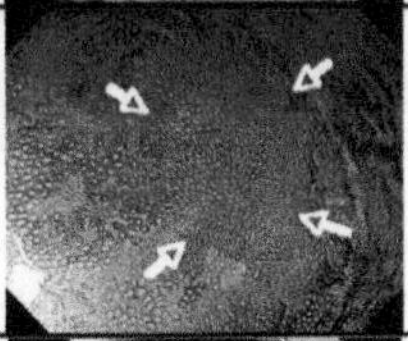	Small tubular or round pits that are smaller than the normal pit	Neoplastic.	Endoscopic.
IIIL	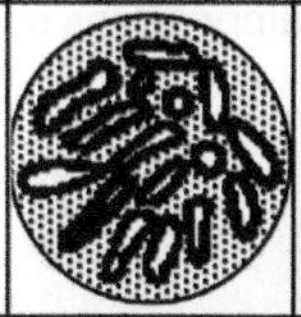	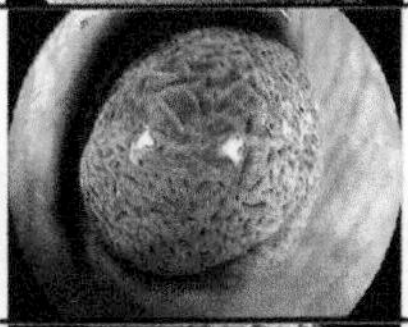	Tubular or roundish pits that are larger than the normal pits.	Neoplastic.	Endoscopic.
IV	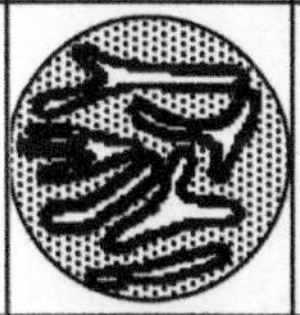	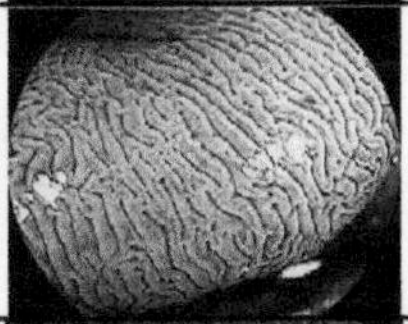	Branch-like or gyrus-like pits.	Neoplastic.	Endoscopic.
VI	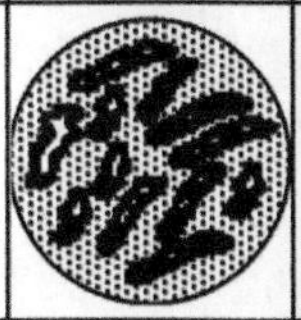		Irregularly arranged pits with type IIIs, IIIL, IV type pit patterns.	Neoplastic (invasive).	Endoscopic or surgical.
VN	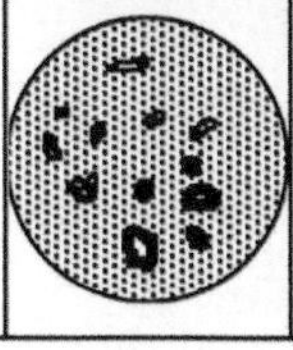	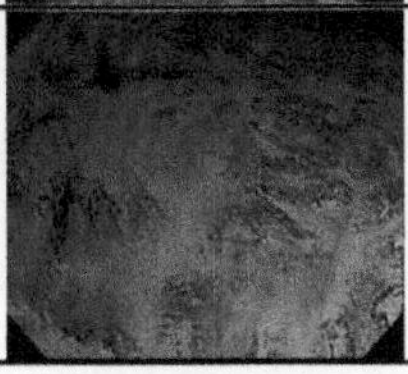	Non-structural pits.	Neoplastic (massive submucosal invasive).	Surgical.

Fig. 37. Current pit-pattern classification of colorectal neoplasms may not be applicable in colitic IBD. The analysis of pit patterns of possible NP-CRN in patients with colitic IBD is difficult for many reasons. Inflammatory activity may mimic neoplasia. The regenerative hyperplastic villous mucosa is difficult to distinguish from neoplastic pit patterns. (*From* Tanaka S, Kaltenbach T, Chayama K, et al. High magnification colonoscopy (with videos). Gastrointest Endosc 2006;64:604–13; with permission.)

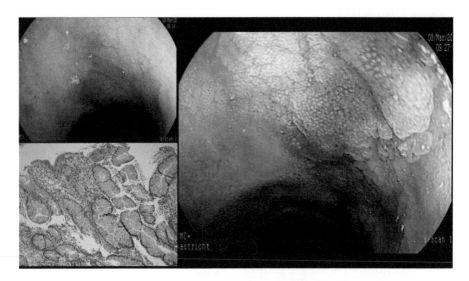

Fig. 38. Inflammatory polyp. High definition imaging enables the endoscopist to discriminate between inflammatory polyps, serrated lesions, and lesions with LGD, HGD, or invasive cancer. It is unnecessary to biopsy or remove obvious inflammatory polyps or lesions, such as seen here.

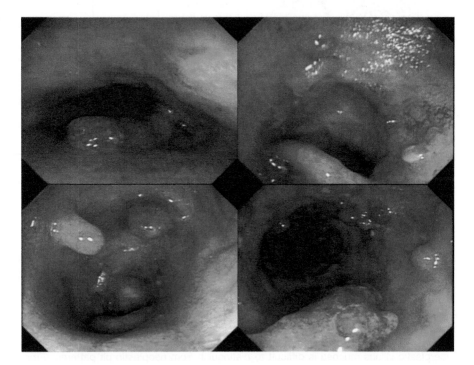

Fig. 39. Biopsies of all suspicious lesions are recommended to exclude dysplasia. This 35-year-old man with an indeterminate colitis had a 1-cm inflammatory-appearing polypoid lesion within a colitic area. Biopsies excluded dysplasia and confirmed chronic inflammation.

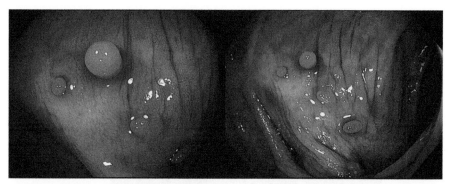

Fig. 40. Inflammatory polyps. In addition to enhancing the border, chromoendoscopy makes it easier to examine the mucosal surface of lesions and facilitates the recognition of inflammatory patterns. Below, a few examples of hyperplastic polyps and sessile serrated adenomas/ polyps are presented.

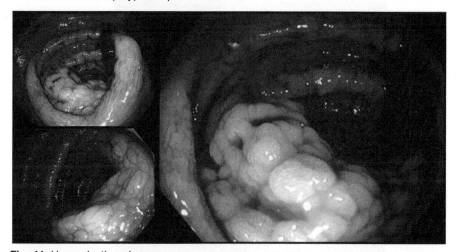

Fig. 41. Hyperplastic polyp.

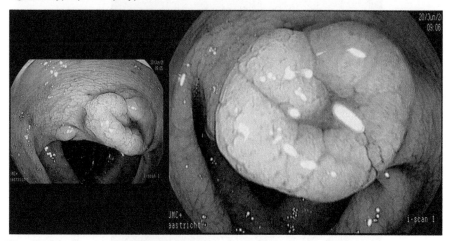

Fig. 42. Sessile serrated adenoma/polyp.

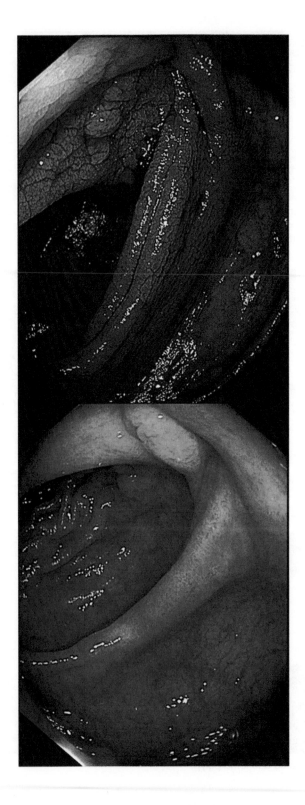

Fig. 43. Sessile serrated adenoma/polyp.

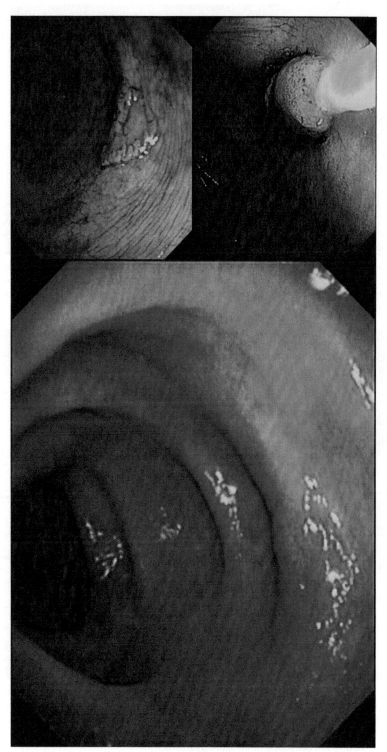

Fig. 44. Depressed neoplasm. Visualization of the depressed morphology required the application of chromoendoscopy. The depressed center of this nonpolypoid (0-IIc) lesion with LGD can only be shown by spraying indigo carmine to show it pooling in the depressed part.

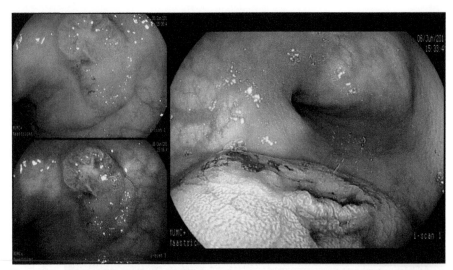

Fig. 45. See above (**Fig. 44**). Visualization of the depressed morphology required the application of chromoendoscopy. It is important to understand that the depressed area likely contains the most advanced histology. Thus, both biopsy can be targeted and removal can be optimized.

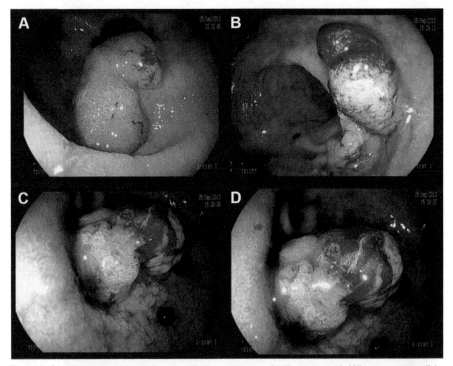

Fig. 46. (*A–D*) Polypoid neoplasms can be endoscopically resected. Whenever possible, lesions less than 2 cm in size should be resected in one piece (ie, en bloc) using EMR. The use of chromoendoscopy can facilitate delineation of the neoplastic borders and ensure complete resection. Following resection, the mucosa around the site should be biopsied to exclude the presence of invisible dysplasia.

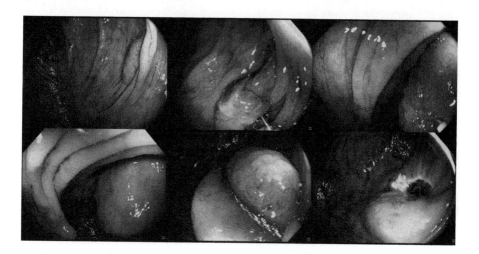

Fig. 47. Dynamic injection can be useful in IBD. Sessile and non-polypoid colorectal lesions in patients with IBD may be best cut after injection. Using the dynamic injection technique the injection is directed into the lumen, to mold the fluid bleb formation. Using slight upward tip deflection, the lumen is suctioned and the needle catheter nominally pulled back while directing the injection into the lumen. In this case, the lesion lifted nicely to form a large bleb. EMR is performed, placing a snare at the normal surrounding edges for en bloc resection. In nonlifting cases, because of underlying fibrosis endoscopic submucosal dissection may be necessary for complete resection.[14]

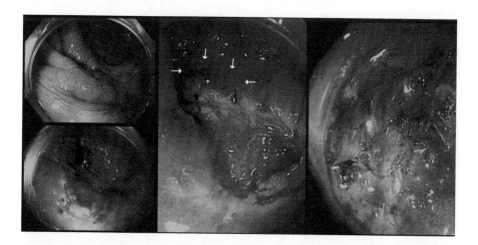

Fig. 48. Ensuring complete resection. Close endoscopic visualization of the surroundings of the resection area to ensure complete resection cannot be overemphasized. In this case, indigo carmine is applied to delineate its borders. EMR is performed, showing significant fibrosis. However, close inspection of the defect borders shows residual lesion (*arrows*). Repeat snare of the site is immediately performed to achieve complete resection. Argon plasma coagulation is then used to coagulate the base and edges of the resection.

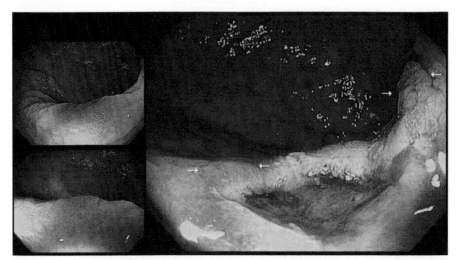

Fig. 49. Evaluation of the surroundings is critical. Following resection, close inspection of the resection defect borders should be performed, and any residual neoplasia removed. In addition, the mucosa around the site should be biopsied to exclude the presence of invisible dysplasia.

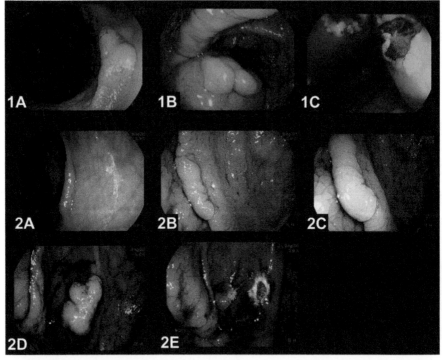

Fig. 50. Multiple nonpolypoid neoplasms can be endoscopically resected during a single procedure. A 62-year-old patient with long-standing Crohn's colitis underwent surveillance colonoscopy that showed multiple neoplasms distributed throughout the colon. (*1A* to *1C*) and (*2A* to *2E*) illustrate details of diagnosis and resection of the lesions. Chromoendoscopy using indigo carmine 0.4% was used for delineation of the borders and examination of the epithelial surface. En bloc EMR resections were performed (*1C, 2E*). Histopathology showed LGD within chronic colitis.

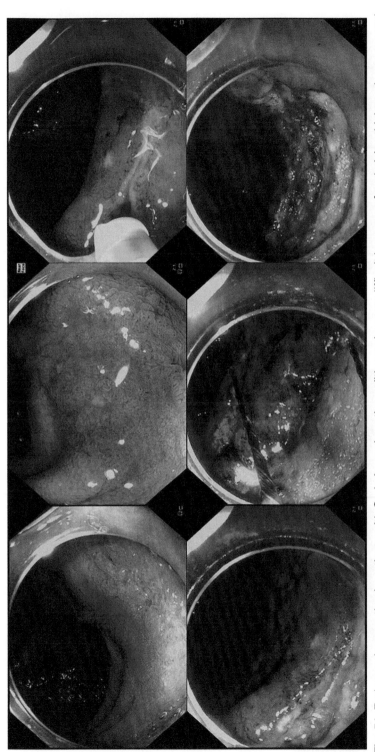

Fig. 51. Endoscopic resection in patients with Crohn's or ulcerative colitis can be very difficult because of underlying thickened mucosa and fibrosis. Multiple biopsies for removal of such lesions must be avoided. EMR is usually the most appropriate endoscopic therapy, noting still the high level of difficulty and risk in endoscopic resection of IBD lesions. Endoscopic submucosal dissection may be necessary for complete resection in some cases, such as shown here. Following injection of the submucosa, there is minimal lifting. Thus, a dual knife is used to make a circumferential incision around the lesion border and dissect the fibrosis submucosally, after which a snare is used to remove the lesion in one piece.

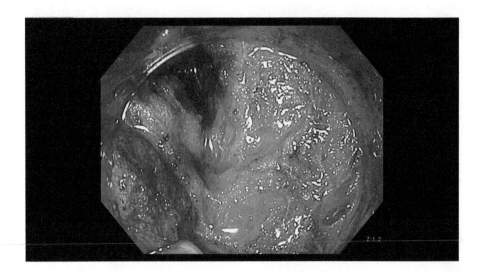

Fig. 52. Severe fibrosis in Crohn's or ulcerative colitis can make endoscopic removal technically difficult. The marked fibrosis of the submucosa of a dysplastic lesion, as shown here during endoscopic submucosal dissection, can lead to the lesion not rising up during endoscopic resection.

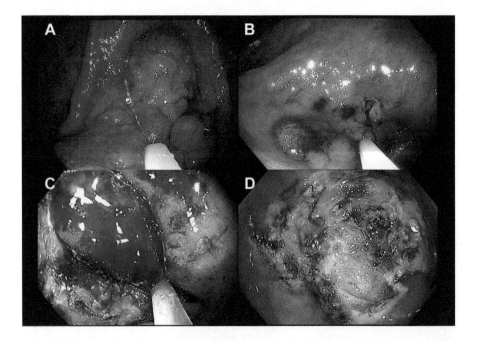

Fig. 53. EMR in the setting of submucosal fibrosis. Resection is this setting is exceedingly difficult and risky. (*A*) The lesion did not lift adequately despite a large amount of injection medium. (*B*) The lesion could not be captured by a snare. (*C*) The cuts were small. (*D*) The underlying fibrosis was exposed.

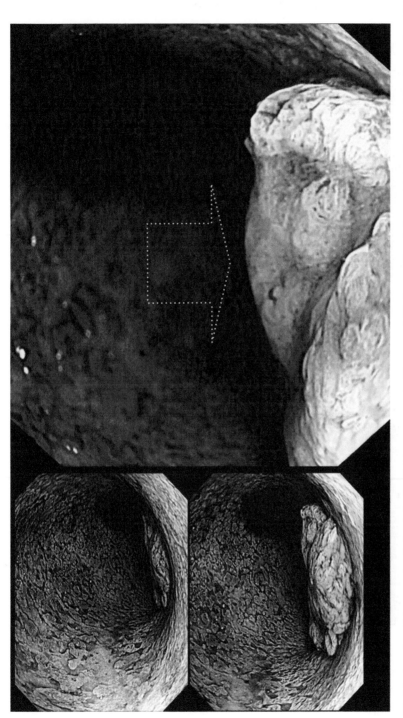

Fig. 54. A lesion should be examined closely to facilitate assessment of its amenability to curative endoscopic resection. On closer inspection, this sessile lesion was considered to have features suspicious for invasive malignancy; that is, the center of the lesion is depressed and the surface is amorphous with loss of mucosal detail. Hence, decisions pertaining to endoscopic versus surgical resection were deferred pending biopsy results. Biopsies should be targeted to the most concerning area of the lesion, as shown here (*arrow*), which confirmed invasive cancer. Surgical resection demonstrated a T1, N0 lesion. (Images courtesy of Professor Shinji Tanaka, Hiroshima University.)

LIMITATIONS OF CHROMOENDOSCOPY

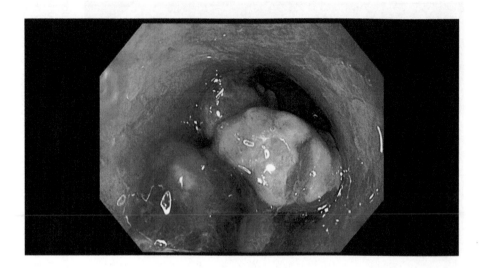

Fig. 55. Random biopsy is still indicated when a large number of pseudopolyps are present. The presence of a large number of postinflammatory polyps may complicate surveillance colonoscopy with chromoendoscopy and targeted biopsy. It is difficult to examine the pseudopolyps and the underlying mucosa when the lumen is filled with the polyps. In such cases, random biopsies are indicated to maximize dysplasia detection.[15]

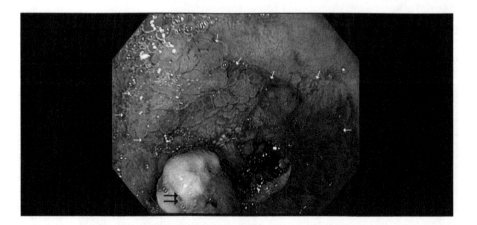

Fig. 56. Dysplasia in the setting of large pseudopolyps. In addition to random biopsy, chromoendoscopy was used in this case. Note the appearance of a superficial elevated lesion (*white arrows*), which on biopsy proved to be HGD, surrounding the polypoid lesion (*double black arrows*).

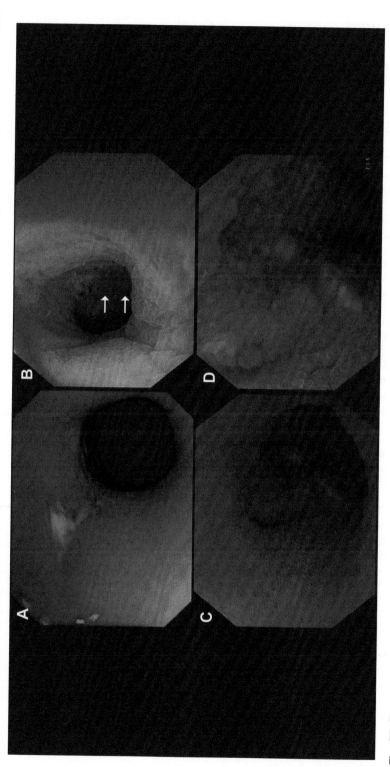

Fig. 57. Examination of a stricture can be difficult because of poor lighting within it, which occurred because of the narrowed lumen. A 79-year-old patient with long-standing ulcerative colitis presented for reevaluation of a stricture in the sigmoid colon. The patient was diagnosed to have the stricture 6 years earlier, but he declined surgery. Over the years, he underwent multiple colonoscopies with biopsies that did not show malignancy (A). The appearance of a cancer within the stricture was finally seen when the stricture was well illuminated (*arrows, B*). The lumen was kept distended using water infusion. On close-up, the lesion appeared neoplastic (C). The center of the lesion (*D*) was suspicious for invasive cancer. Biopsy showed invasive adenocarcinoma. Patients with ulcerative colitis are recommended to have surgery when a colonic stricture is found.

ACKNOWLEDGEMENTS

The authors thank Drs. Shinji Tanaka, Ronald Yeh, and Hazem Hammad for their generous contributions.

REFERENCES

1. Wang YR, Cangemi JR, Loftus EV Jr, et al. Rate of early/missed colorectal cancers after colonoscopy in older patients with or without inflammatory bowel disease in the United States. Am J Gastroenterol 2013;108:444–9.
2. Soetikno R, Subramanian V, Kaltenbach T, et al. The detection of nonpolypoid (flat and depressed) colorectal neoplasms in patients with inflammatory bowel disease. Gastroenterology 2013;144:1349–52, 1352.e1–6.
3. Jaramillo E, Watanabe M, Befrits R, et al. Small, flat colorectal neoplasias in long-standing ulcerative colitis detected by high-resolution electronic video endoscopy. Gastrointest Endosc 1996;44:15–22.
4. Rutter MD, Saunders BP, Wilkinson KH, et al. Most dysplasia in ulcerative colitis is visible at colonoscopy. Gastrointest Endosc 2004;60:334–9.
5. Sanchez-Yague A, Kaltenbach T, Yamamoto H, et al. The endoscopic cap that can (with videos). Gastrointest Endosc 2012;76:169–78.e1–2.
6. Matsuda T, Parra-Blanco A, Saito Y, et al. Assessment of likelihood of submucosal invasion in non-polypoid colorectal neoplasms. Gastrointest Endosc Clin N Am 2010;20:487–96.
7. The Paris endoscopic classification of superficial neoplastic lesions: esophagus, stomach and colon. Gastrointest Endosc 2003;58:S3–43.
8. Yasutomi M, Baba S, Hojo K, et al. Japanese classification of colorectal carcinoma. Tokyo: Kanehara & Co, LTD; 1997.
9. Laine L, Barkun A, Kaltenbach T, et al. Surveillance for colorectal endoscopic neoplasia detection and management in inflammatory bowel disease patients: International Consensus recommendations. San Francisco (CA): 2014.
10. Subramanian V, Ramappa V, Telakis E, et al. Comparison of high definition with standard white light endoscopy for detection of dysplastic lesions during surveillance colonoscopy in patients with colonic inflammatory bowel disease. Inflamm Bowel Dis 2013;19:350–5.
11. Picco MF, Pasha S, Leighton JA, et al. Procedure time and the determination of polypoid abnormalities with experience: implementation of a chromoendoscopy program for surveillance colonoscopy for ulcerative colitis. Inflamm Bowel Dis 2013;19:1913–20.
12. Ignjatovic A, East JE, Subramanian V, et al. Narrow band imaging for detection of dysplasia in colitis: a randomized controlled trial. Am J Gastroenterol 2012;107:885–90.
13. van den Broek FJ, Fockens P, van Eeden S, et al. Narrow-band imaging versus high-definition endoscopy for the diagnosis of neoplasia in ulcerative colitis. Endoscopy 2011;43:108–15.
14. Soetikno R, Kaltenbach T. Dynamic submucosal injection technique. Gastrointest Endosc Clin N Am 2010;20:497–502.
15. Party CCACSW. Clinical Practice Guidelines for Surveillance Colonoscopy - in adenoma follow-up; following curative resection of colorectal cancer; and for cancer surveillance in inflammatory bowel disease. Cancer Council Australia; 2011.

Index

Note: Page numbers of article titles are in **boldface** type.

A

B

C

Gastrointest Endoscopy Clin N Am 24 (2014) 521–526
http://dx.doi.org/10.1016/S1052-5157(14)00050-6
1052-5157/14/$ – see front matter © 2014 Elsevier Inc. All rights reserved.

giendo.theclinics.com

Printed and bound by CPI Group (UK) Ltd, Croydon, CR0 4YY

03/10/2024

01040486-0001